THE ART OF WAR
on
Dental Health

Margaret McMillan

BALBOA.
PRESS
A DIVISION OF HAY HOUSE

Balboa Press books may be ordered through booksellers or by contacting:

Balboa Press
A Division of Hay House
1663 Liberty Drive
Bloomington, IN 47403
www.balboapress.com
1 (877) 407-4847

Because of the dynamic nature of the Internet, any web addresses or
links contained in this book may have changed since publication and
may no longer be valid. The views expressed in this work are solely those
of the author and do not necessarily reflect the views of the publisher,
and the publisher hereby disclaims any responsibility for them.

The author of this book does not dispense medical advice or prescribe the use
of any technique as a form of treatment for physical, emotional, or medical
problems without the advice of a physician, either directly or indirectly. The
intent of the author is only to offer information of a general nature to help you
in your quest for emotional and spiritual well-being. In the event you use any
of the information in this book for yourself, which is your constitutional right,
the author and the publisher assume no responsibility for your actions.

Any people depicted in stock imagery provided by Thinkstock are models,
and such images are being used for illustrative purposes only.
Certain stock imagery © Thinkstock.

Printed in the United States of America.

ISBN: 978-1-4525-1555-7 (sc)
ISBN: 978-1-4525-1557-1 (hc)
ISBN: 978-1-4525-1556-4 (e)

Library of Congress Control Number: 2014909577

Balboa Press rev. date: 10/29/2014

CONTENTS

· · · · · · · · · · · · · · · · · · · ·

LIST OF ILLUSTRATIONS

· · · · · · · · · · · · · · · · · · · ·

"The soft overcomes the hard. The slow overcome the fast. Let your working remain a mystery. Just show people the results."
TAO TE CHING

PREFACE

"Tis skill, not strength, that governs the ship."
THOMAS FULLER

As a child I had crooked teeth and a serious overbite, and orthodontics was not yet a specialty. Dentists who were already performing in this field had been grandfathered in as specialists. The doctor on whom my mouth depended for repair was a gruff older man. He tapped the bands onto my teeth with a mallet and shoved my teeth apart to get the bands in place. Hurting, I closed my eyes as tears rolled down my cheeks. The next thing I knew I was picked up by the collar and shoved back into the chair, admonished with, "Stop your crying!" Until that moment I didn't even realize I was crying.

For years after that experience, I had a difficult time sitting in a dental chair. I knew, even then, that it should not hurt that badly, and I decided I wanted to be a dentist so I could prove myself right.

When I was a high school sophomore, our class received an assignment to write an essay on what we wished to be when we grew up, including research on that career. I chose dentist. I got a B because, as the teacher said, "the research is good, but this is unrealistic. Girls become hygienists, not dentists." Two years later, the dental hygiene school accepted me. I attended with a full-on attitude against it.

Fortunately, one of my faculty advisors, Dolores Ickis, pulled me aside one day and asked why my grades were so poor. (I got C's by failing midterm exams and then acing the finals.) I told the professor, "I do not want to be a hygienist. I want to be a dentist, so I don't bother studying."

To this day I cherish her comment: "One day they will accept girls into dental school, and they are going to look at these grades. You need to show them you are capable of getting A's."

I did.

It took four years of applying to dental schools, but I finally got accepted to, and graduated with honors from, Northwestern University Dental School. In the past couple decades since then, I've heard every reason and horror story imaginable for why people believe they have poor dental health.

My awareness of the fact that "you don't know what you don't know" sent me on a quest to study health, especially how it relates to the mouth and the teeth.

Helping others increase their knowledge of their overall health, especially dental health, became the reason I decided to write this book—to help you learn how you can and should keep your teeth in your mouth for a lifetime.

Sun Tzu was a general and a legend in ancient China; he won more battles than any other battalion leader of his time. Prior to Sun Tzu's retirement, the king asked him to write down how he won almost every time. Sun Tzu knew his subject so well that his advice resonates to this day, not only on the battlefield, but also in dealing with everyday challenges.

Sun Tzu's *The Art of War* offers relevant and analogous advice on winning battles, or at least how to keep losses to a minimum, and provides lessons applicable to seeking and maintaining good health, which is a daily battle.

I hope in following the instructions in this book that you, too, can keep your losses to a minimum and win the battle against dental disease so that your overall health improves. My goal as a dentist is to become a prevention-only based practice, barring emergencies. I hope, like Sun Tzu, to be a winning general dentist.

ACKNOWLEDGMENTS

· · · · · · · · · · · · · · · · · · · ·

*"First say to yourself what you would be, then
do what you have to do to be it."*
EPICTETUS

Having attended Northwestern University Dental School in the early 1980s, I was blessed to attend a school associated with some of the pioneers in the evolution of dental education. Dr. G. V. Black learned dentistry at an early age in the mid-1800s, and he made a career studying how cavities form. He classified the teeth and developed a system for restoring them to a healthy state. Referred to as the father of modern dentistry, Dr. Black was instrumental in founding formal dental education and promoting dentistry as a profession. In 1896, Dr. Black became the first dean of Northwestern University Dental School.

Dr. L. D. Pankey, a dental education pioneer from the 1930s to the 1980s, made it his life's purpose to not only educate doctors in technical proficiency, but also encourage a balance between work, home, and spiritual life. Dr. Pankey championed the philosophy, "Teeth do not walk into my office," and he educated patients on the importance of keeping their teeth healthy. While a student at Northwestern, I had the privilege of receiving clinical instruction from Dr. Pankey. I still attend continuing education seminars at the dental learning center named for him, the Pankey Institute, in Key Biscayne, Florida. Dr. Pankey's philosophy of care greatly informs my own.

Dr. Peter Dawson, one of Dr. Pankey's key students at the Institute, also taught at Northwestern during my tenure there. He, too, developed a center for higher dental education, the Dawson Academy, that I still attend for continuing education in St. Petersburg, Florida. Dr. Dawson's instruction helped me fully embrace how important the jaw is to the teeth, and vice versa.

At the Pankey Institute I had the privilege of learning under Dr. Pankey's successor, Dr. Irwin Becker, who instilled in me the importance of maintaining a balanced life between home and work and never settling for "good enough."

Dr. Terry Tanaka of the University of Southern California Dental School lectures worldwide. While attending one of his lectures, he noticed my jaw discrepancy and asked if I suffered lower back pain. (I do.) His astuteness inspired me to pursue a master's level of continuing dental education so I can help people understand, like he did for me, how the health of the teeth and jaw influence the rest of the body.

Ms. Dolores Ickis, one of my instructors in the dental hygiene program at Prairie State College in Chicago Heights, Illinois, was the first person to validate my desire to become a dentist and inspired in me an unquenchable thirst for learning.

One of my dearest friends, Dr. J. Michael Major, a published author himself, has always had kind and encouraging words to lift my spirits when no one else can.

Bob and Darlene McMillan, my mom and dad, instilled in me a strong sense of perseverance and integrity, allowing me to pursue my dreams in spite of the odds stacked against me.

My husband, Slava Kuznetsov, always brings joy to my soul and gives wonderful ideas to add flavor to all my stories.

My most gracious thanks go to my editor, Martha Goudey, for taking me down the path from crazy idea to published book. Without Martha's input and keen eye for detail, I would still be floundering in ideas.

INTRODUCTION

. . . .

"A man who is always ready to believe what is told to him will never do well, especially a business man."
PETRONIUS

In approximately 500 BC, the king of Wu, Ho Lu, asked Sun Tzu before he retired to write down how he became the most winning general ever. The story goes something like this, modernized in my translation:

Ho Lu read the manuscript and dared Sun Tzu to a test by asking him if his theory would work even with (heaven forbid) women. Sun Tzu took on the challenge, knowing his theory well.

One hundred and eighty ladies of the king's court were brought from the palace, and Sun Tzu divided them into two teams, each led by the king's favorite concubines. He asked them all if they knew left from right. When they said yes, he ordered them *"Right face!"*

The ladies broke out in giggles.

Sun Tzu stated that if words are not clear and understood, the general is to be blamed.

He took the time to teach them right and left, forward and backward, and again gave the order, *"Right face!"*

Again, the ladies giggled.

This time Sun Tzu said that if the words are not clear, the general is to blame, but if the orders are clear and the soldiers disobey anyway, the officers shoulder the blame.

He then ordered the king's favorite concubines, the leaders, beheaded. Ho Lu did not like that one bit and ordered Sun Tzu to stop the demonstration.

Sun Tzu replied that he could not stop, as he was on the battlefield now, with a job to finish. He said that his majesty had ordered a job to be done, and now that he was in the middle of it, he must continue.

The beheading took place.

Sun Tzu appointed the next two in line as the new leaders and ordered, *"Right face!"* Every lady turned to the right in unison and completed every maneuver with precision and accuracy.

Sun Tzu then informed King Ho Lu that he would be completely safe from invasion now, as even his ladies were fully prepared for battle.

The story of Sun Tzu is not meant to cause you to fear I shall behead any patient who won't listen to me. Most people are already afraid of the dentist as it is. My goal is to provide you with tools and information necessary to achieve and maintain good dental health, and as a result, overall health. Teeth are not only a part of your body, but they are essential to sound health. In turn, every aspect of your health, including physical and emotional well-being, plays a part in achieving dental health. You may be surprised to learn about certain health issues you may never have attributed to dental disease, such as lower back pain or migraine headaches. You may surprise yourself when considering past decisions, such as "It's only a back tooth—just pull it."

An animal in the wild dies if it loses its teeth. You have the fortunate advantage of dentistry to help you preserve your teeth. If you have had serious health and dental issues in the past, this book is for you to use to regain health and take control of your life again.

Sun Tzu wrote 13 chapters for *The Art of War*. I have taken artistic liberty with these chapters to use them to explain how to achieve tooth and gum health, and as a result, overall health. It is time to declare war on poor health. Let's start with teeth.

"She laughs at everything you say. Why? Because she has fine teeth."
BENJAMIN FRANKLIN

CHAPTER 1

. . . .

THE LAYING OF PLANS

"Hair is the first thing. And teeth the second. Hair and teeth. A man got those two things he's got it all."
JAMES BROWN

Understanding Your Mouth

Sun Tzu said the art of war is a matter of life and death, a road to either safety or ruin, and it can on no account be neglected. The same rule applies to health. Neglected, one dies. Now, we're all going to die anyway, but living a full life to a ripe old age beats the heck out of taking dozens of pills daily, with constant trips to the hospital for pain or other suffering, until we die. Learning what constitutes good health begins by knowing what "healthy" looks like.

The mouth seems to be a simple organ when, in fact, it is the most complex organ in contact with the outside world. Quick to adapt to change, rapidly healed when injured, self-cleansing (with proper diet and tooth alignment), and the center of social activities, the mouth shows emotion, allows communication, aids in lovemaking, nourishes the body, cleanses the digestive tract, helps fight off bacterial or viral invaders, and—best of all—feeds us, giving us the energy needed to survive.

The human mouth consists of a jaw, the muscles that support and work it, cheeks, bones, a tongue, teeth, and the passage leading to other areas where food is digested or air is breathed. Let's begin with the teeth and the many ways they function as a whole.

The adult human mouth houses thirty-two teeth. Young children have twenty teeth, and children between the ages of five and fourteen have any number between twenty and twenty-eight. When a person is between sixteen and twenty-two years old, his or her wisdom teeth start to come in. This book will explain the importance of baby teeth; however, for now I will focus on the adult mouth.

The first thing almost everyone notices when meeting another person is the mouth. A beautiful smile is one of the most attractive aspects of a human. Although a smile may be warm and inviting, without the teeth it loses its luster. Personally, I'm not attracted to the excessive whiteness glaring at us today, but I do notice a bright, healthy smile from quite a distance away. Smiles speak in every language and in nearly every species. Smile at the gorilla in the zoo, and watch him smile right back at you.

Teeth also contour and help shape the face. Each tooth root has a distinctive shape and size, encased in bone. Tooth loss causes this boney encasement to dissolve and disappear. Molar roots, especially the six-year molar, splay widely and have thick contours. When extracted, the bone housing these roots shrinks, causing the cheekbone to collapse. Missing bicuspids collapse the cheek just under the nose. Missing canines and incisors cave in the entire lip area. Picture the face of a person with no teeth. Notice the collapsed bone? Even one missing tooth causes a change in facial contour.

Teeth affect your speech. Remember when all you wanted for "Chrithmath" was your two front "teef"? The *f, l, m, s, th,* and *v* sounds depend on the tooth-lip, tongue-tooth position, or the free air space between top and bottom teeth. When I make a denture or do any kind of "smile makeover" for a patient, I put the individual through elaborate phonetic exercises. Before I complete the denture process, I assess the pronunciation, lip placement, and overall facial measurements during speech to ensure I place the teeth properly according to the patient's anatomy. Think of someone you know who suddenly speaks with a click or whistle or slur. Provided the person is sober, he or she probably received new teeth in the wrong position, where the new teeth infringe upon the muscle movements or airflow for proper speech.

Professional singers and speakers notice this immediately. The muscular forces of the lips and tongue determine where your teeth place themselves in the arches. We call this the "neutral zone." The muscles keep the teeth in harmony. Harmony and form are essential to proper functioning of the teeth and jaws. If the muscle is not correct, the teeth will not be stable.

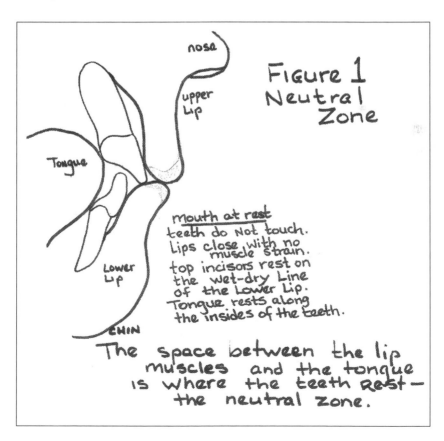

nose

upper lip

FIGURE 1
Neutral
Zone

Tongue

Lower lip

CHIN

mouth at rest
teeth do not touch.
Lips close with no
muscle strain.
top incisors rest on
the wet-dry line
of the lower lip.
Tongue rests along
the insides of the teeth.

The space between the lip
muscles and the tongue
is where the teeth rest —
the neutral zone.

Form follows function in all of your body. If you injure your knee and walk with a limp long enough, you will alter the alignment of your spine from the excess muscle pull on one side. It is the same with your jaw and teeth. The cheek and tongue muscles keep the teeth in perfect alignment, which aids in perfect speech—regardless of the language spoken. Infringe on that space, and the muscles fight to get it back or adapt to work differently.

Finally, the most important function of teeth is to chew food. Wild animals die when they lose teeth because they can no longer eat. Humans have dentistry, as well as blenders: dentistry to prevent loss, blenders to make chewing easier once tooth loss has occurred. As you will learn in later chapters, good nutrition and proper digestion begin in the mouth.

To help you fully comprehend the importance of chewing food properly, I will first identify each tooth and its individual function. The first year in dental school, students must identify a single tooth from a pile of miscellaneous teeth and must carve in wax each tooth individually to precision. Right, left, top, and bottom teeth each have their own unique markings based on the functions they perform. Again, form follows function.

There are four types of teeth: incisors, canines, bicuspids, and molars. The four big front top teeth seen in your smile and the four tiny teeth below them in the lower jaw are your incisors. If you draw a line directly down the middle of your face, separating the right and left sides of the face, you create a mirror image of the two right and two left incisors. Their shape mimics that of the face, being ovoid, round, square, or trapezoid.

The two front teeth are called the central incisors, and the ones on the side are the lateral incisors. The length of the top central incisors is exactly one-sixteenth the length of your face when measuring from the top of the forehead to the chin, and the width

4

of the central incisors is exactly one-sixteenth the distance from cheek edge to cheek edge.

The edge of the upper central incisors is almost flat across, with a slightly rounded corner on the side away from the middle of the face. The lip side of the incisors is smooth and arcs ever so slightly outward from gum edge to biting edge. The tongue side caves inward and has a lump just above the gum edge to stop the bottom incisors from biting any deeper. This not only protects the roof of the mouth from being cut into, but also protects the back teeth from the force of the jaw muscles.

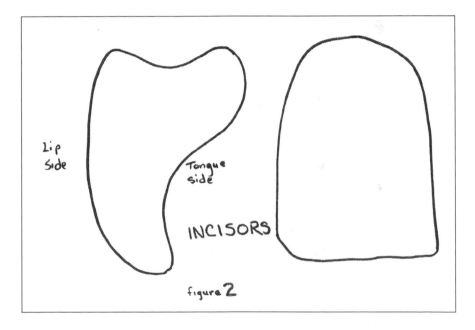

Lip
Side

Tongue
side

INCISORS

figure 2

The lateral incisors are slightly shorter in length and width than the central incisors, and they are a bit rounder in all aspects. All incisors have flat edges. The four lower incisors tuck under the top teeth as the jaw closes, to act as a pair of scissors. As their name implies, their function is to incise—or cut—food into a small enough bite to fit into the mouth for proper chewing.

When the jaw comes forward and the incisors meet edge to edge, the top central incisors ride flat on the lower central incisors and part of the lower lateral incisors. This guides the jaw into proper alignment during certain chewing movements, which is known as "anterior guidance." Along with the canines, this prevents the back teeth from slamming into each other. When the front teeth are worn or broken away, the back teeth lose this protection.

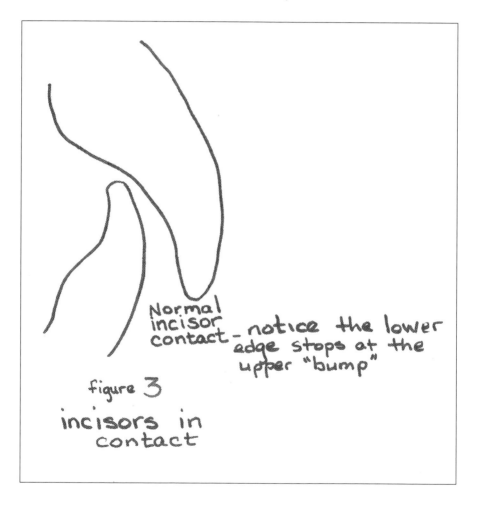

Normal incisor contact – notice the lower edge stops at the upper "bump"

figure 3
incisors in contact

The canines in the upper jaw lie directly under the pupil of the eye when looking straight ahead, hence the nickname "eye teeth." The edge comes to a point, known as a cusp, and therefore the proper dental term is the *cuspid*. The roots are very long and thick, and they end just under the area of the eye that houses the nerves and blood vessels that lead to the eye. Both upper and lower canines possess the longest and strongest roots in that area of the mouth because they function as the cornerstone to the teeth. When the jaw moves left or right, the lower canines glide along the underbelly of the upper canines to separate the back teeth until the central incisors can place the jaw into the proper position. (Note: This is impossible to duplicate in dentures because both sides of the plastic teeth must be in full contact at all times to remain stable and not pop out when chewing.) This guidance allows the teeth to separate food and process it backward toward the throat, as well as to prevent the back teeth from shearing each other off. When grinding one's teeth wears the canines down, these protective mechanisms can no longer function. The back teeth will begin to break.

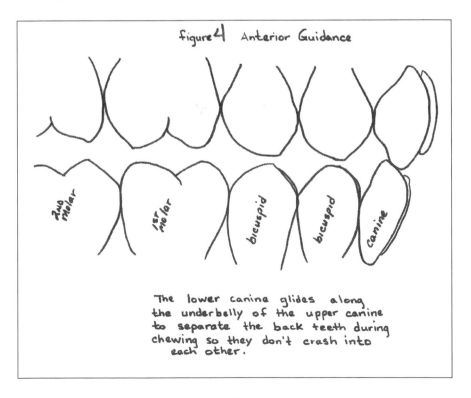

figure 4 Anterior Guidance

2nd molar
1st molar
bicuspid
bicuspid
canine

The lower canine glides along the underbelly of the upper canine to separate the back teeth during chewing so they don't crash into each other.

When it comes to eating, the canines grab the food and hold it still while the incisors cut it off to be placed into the mouth. If you ever bite into a sandwich and the bread readily breaks off but the lettuce stays whole and is not torn off by the teeth, your canines and incisors do not function properly.

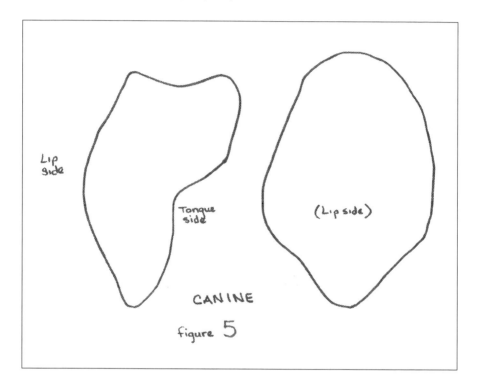

Lip side

Tongue side

(Lip side)

CANINE

figure 5

Directly behind the canines lie two teeth per quadrant that have two points (cusps) on them. Commonly known as bicuspids, dentists call them premolars because they look like skinny, tiny, narrow molars. Aside from brightening the grin of those who emulate Julia Roberts' smile, bicuspids serve a small but critical job. The two cusps form a sluiceway so food can sluice—or be pushed backward—to the molars.

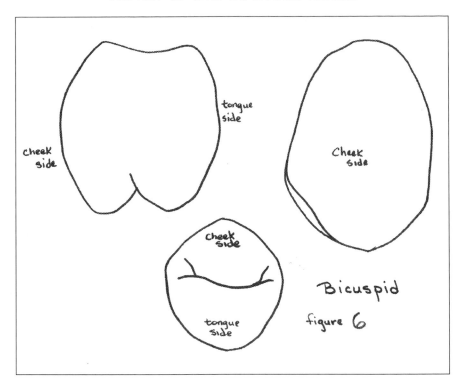

tongue side

cheek side

Cheek Side

Cheek Side

tongue side

Bicuspid

figure 6

When erupting into the mouth, the roots of the baby molars guide the bicuspids into place. A child's mouth does not need the extra sluiceway, so there are no baby bicuspids. The baby molar roots are broad and curvy to enable the bicuspid to be placed properly.

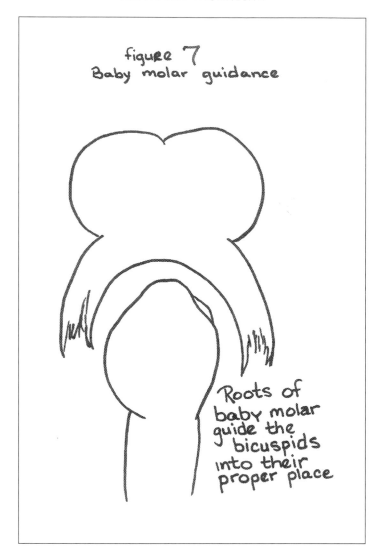

figuℝe 7
Baby molar guidance

Roots of baby molar guide the bicuspids into their proper place

And now, the molars: the most important teeth in the mouth and the most neglected. We chew food with our molars. Without molars, you cannot chew food properly. That is worth repeating because when people have problems with molars, many opt to have them pulled rather than treated. I cannot count how often I have heard, "Oh, it's just a back tooth—pull it."

Molars possess three, four, or five cusps and have a large table for food to sit upon. The upper molars overlap the lower molars to hold the cheeks out of the way as the jaw closes, crushing the teeth together and intertwining the cusps to mash the food. Think of how a zipper works. The zipper teeth intertwine into each other to lock closed. Get your skin caught in between these teeth, and *ouch!* This mechanism works the same for our teeth. The food gets stuck between the upper and lower cusps of the molars, mashing it. Get your cheek caught in between the teeth, and *ouch!*

Humans have three molars per quadrant of the mouth (upper right, upper left, lower right, and lower left). The first one in each quadrant erupts into your mouth when you reach six years of age. The first adult teeth to erupt in the mouth and before any baby teeth fall out are the six-year molars (also called the first molars). They enter directly behind the baby molars and maintain a space to properly hold the correct position so that the other teeth erupt correctly. Strong and healthy baby teeth, properly cared for, allow the six-year molar to come in straight and not move forward, allowing for all the other teeth to follow suit. You can now understand the most important reason to keep baby teeth healthy. The first molar sidles up to the baby molars and maintains a strong position there to guide the bite. The baby molar roots guide the bicuspids up directly next to the molars. Lose a baby molar before the bicuspids are ready to erupt, or worse, before the first molar comes in, and the entire adult tooth lineup breaks down.

This first molar encompasses the largest area of the mouth. Big, strong, wide, and thick, it crushes food.

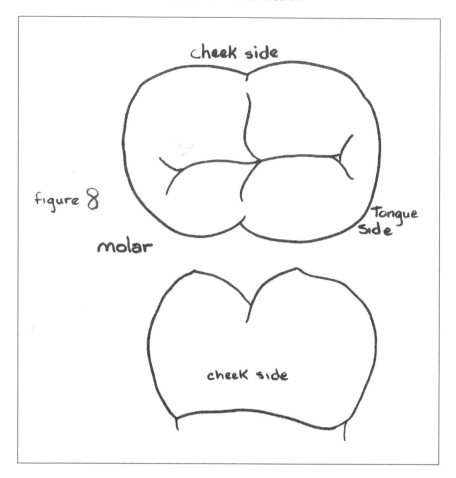

figure 8

molar

cheek side

Tongue Side

cheek side

The second molar erupts into the mouth at about twelve years old, right behind the first molar. Other than the wisdom teeth, this completes the adult dentition. The second molar generally maintains a smaller table, has fewer cusps, and is shorter and rounder than the first molar due to its closeness to the "hinge" of the "door"—the jaw joint. When you slam your fingers in a door, it hurts. When you get your fingers caught in the space by the hinges, you can lose your fingers. The closer an object is to the hinges, the more damage done. Due to their location, second molars tend to break easily when the bite changes. Anterior guidance or the shearing forces of the teeth can be altered during abnormal chewing, such as the horrific habit of grinding teeth. Second molars aid in spreading the chewing forces of food more evenly.

Wisdom teeth, or third molars, were crucial to chewing before McDonald's and processed foods became the norm. Over the generations, many people got Dad's teeth inside Mom's jaw, or genetically the wisdom teeth took the path of Great-Great-Grandpa's. They exhibit all shapes and sizes, sometimes much larger than the first molars, sometimes tinier than the bicuspids. Sometimes they do not form at all. Sometimes they get stuck in the bone or under the second molar and cannot erupt into the mouth.

An impacted tooth is one that is stuck and cannot come into its proper place. When wisdom teeth become impacted, problems can occur much later in life. Cysts, severe cavities, or gum problems can develop on the wisdom tooth or even on the second molar. Under these circumstances, they should be removed. Healing from these extractions occurs far easier in the younger bone, hence the reason many doctors advocate getting them pulled at eighteen years old.

Many differing opinions arise on pulling wisdom teeth, but generally, if they pose no future threat to the integrity of other teeth or your overall health, you can leave them be. But to compromise and potentially lose the second molar tragically decreases the surface area necessary for proper chewing. Molars chew. The more surface area present, the better you can chew, and therefore the better digestion you have.

If you take your time to chew properly and not wolf down your food, that is.

The cellular makeup of all teeth is identical, and it is similar to the makeup of your long bones. The part of the tooth you see in your mouth is called the crown, and the part that anchors it to the bone is called the root. The nerve enters the tooth from the bottom of the root deep within the jaw. The root anchors to the bone with millions of tiny nerve fibers embedded within the bone and the root covering. The root covering is called the cementum and these fibers "cement" the tooth into the bone. When you have a root canal, the doctor removes the nerve entering from the bottom of the tooth. The nerves anchoring the tooth to the bone remain untouched. They function to keep the tooth aware of any potential danger. Their sensitivity is so strong they can feel the presence of a hair between your teeth so you will not crush your teeth together. These nerve fibers pay acute attention to ensure that the teeth do not touch each other unnecessarily or that nothing interferes with their proper contact when necessary. The only time it's necessary for teeth to contact each other is the final act in swallowing, when the lips seal the mouth closed and the tongue pushes the bolus of food down the throat.

Think about this a second. You chew ice cubes. I absolutely do *not* recommend this, but many people chew ice. You crush the cube in half, and your jaw instantly opens so quickly you don't realize it. These fibers amazingly and constantly prevent your teeth from slamming into each other.

Enamel covers the crown of the tooth and makes your teeth appear white. More than 104 shades of tooth color have been classified in dentistry. Enamel, however, is transparent. Think of plastic food wrap. A single sheet is transparent, but when you look at the entire roll, it is white. So it is with enamel. The thicker your enamel (provided it remains undamaged from antibiotics or other growth interferences while it develops), the whiter and stronger your teeth.

Enamel is the strongest living structure known to man. Diamond is the strongest nonliving structure. Diamonds cut enamel, but nothing else truly can. Enamel survives airplane crashes, and bodies are identified using dental records. The only way enamel can be destroyed is with acid or shearing forces of destruction. A very thin film, called a pellicle, covers your teeth naturally to protect enamel from salivary acids. Shearing forces occur when two objects bang into each other at an angle. The cusps and edges of teeth are not designed to withstand angle forces like grinding your teeth.

The main bulk of the tooth, the core strength and cushion, is called dentin. Dentin provides the bulky strength under the enamel to cushion it from the crushing forces of chewing. Dentin also cushions the nerve from traumatic forces in both the crown and the root. Dentin has a yellowish to yellow-brown color, which is what gives teeth their ivory hue.

The nerve likes to have a certain amount of space between it and the cementum or enamel surface. Because of the forces used daily in natural chewing and speech, dentin constantly works to maintain the integrity of the teeth. When compromised, dentin must build a new layer of wall to protect the nerve. Cavities, drilling teeth, breaking teeth, grinding teeth, habits of chewing nonfood substances like pens and bobby pins, and an improper biting force all compromise the dentin's protection for the nerve. The nerve knows only one response to compromise—pain. Whether the sensation is hot, cold, improper biting, drilling, cavity, whatever, the nerve responds with pain. When dentin builds a new wall of protection reinstating the width of protection the nerve likes, the nerve becomes quiet again and all is well. When the trauma occurs too fast or for too long, the dentin cannot keep up, and the nerve gives up and dies. That hurts. That's when you call and beg for a root canal.

Much the same as skin covers muscle and bones, gums cover the bone inside of your mouth and protect the area around the bone and teeth. The gums protecting the teeth like to be only about two or three millimeters deep from where you see the gumline and where the gums actually attach to the tooth, similar to the space where you see the edge of your fingernail and the quick. The gums have a distinct color, the same coral pink as the rest of the mouth tissues, including the tongue, although some ethnic groups may have darker pigmentations. The color of healthy gums matches the exact color of the rest of the mouth tissues.

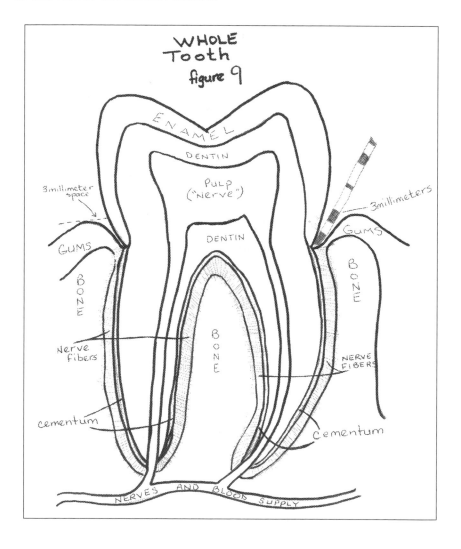

The texture of the gums looks and feels like an orange peel. The gums encircle the top edges, the necks of the teeth, and one can actually draw a straight line from the neck of the tooth all the way through that arch.

Gums completely fill the space between the teeth, forming an almost perfect triangle. Drawing a line across the entire arch from the point of each triangle creates a parallel line to the one drawn at the top of the gums along the neck of the teeth. These two lines are also parallel to the biting and chewing edges of the teeth, as well as to an imaginary line drawn across your pupils when looking straight ahead and parallel to the floor (see Figure 10).

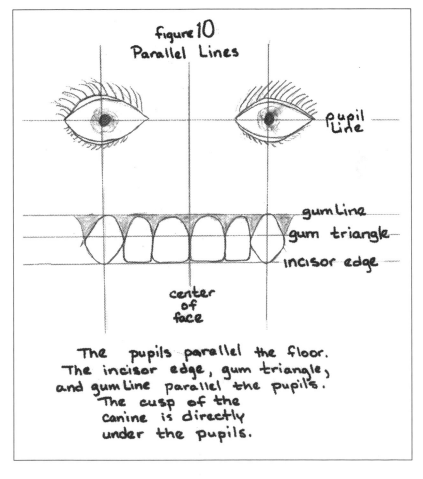

figure 10
Parallel Lines

pupil line

gum line
gum triangle
incisor edge

center of face

The pupils parallel the floor.
The incisor edge, gum triangle, and gum line parallel the pupils.
The cusp of the canine is directly under the pupils.

For the most part, the function of the gums is to protect and give nourishment to the bone and teeth via the many nerves and blood vessels circulating within the gums.

The tongue is the strongest muscle in the body—just ask any dental assistant whose job it is to keep the tongue away from the drill bits. Some patients move their tongue so much it takes two hands and the entire bodily force of the assistant to hold it away from the drill. Taste buds, nerves, blood vessels, and lymph glands are embedded in the body of the tongue. The job of the tongue, aside from speech production, is to push the food (with help from the cheeks) up onto the molar table for chewing, then take that chewed food and push it backward down the throat for proper swallowing. The color of a healthy tongue mimics the exact color of all the internal mouth tissues: coral pink with a slight shininess to it. The texture is smooth, with no cracks, teeth marks, or ulcerations, and the taste bud papillae can be clearly seen.

The uvula (that thingy hanging down in the back of the throat), the tonsils, and the vocal cords all have the same coral pink color, and they all provide a passageway for food to go down and for air to go in and out of the body. The lips close to form a vacuum in swallowing so food travels one direction only. Flaps of tissue close the air passageway to swallow, and others close the food passageway for air to enter and exit the body. Each has its own job, and you never need to think about making one or the other work. But if you are laughing, talking, or breathing heavily while chewing, the flaps can get confused, forcing food down the "wrong pipe." This can be extremely dangerous, even leading to choking and death.

And then there is an often-neglected aspect within the mouth, saliva. Saliva serves many functions. Saliva keeps the teeth wet, neutralizes acids produced by fermenting bacteria, and washes food remnants from the teeth and gums. Saliva wets food so it travels down the pipes into the stomach smoothly, begins the breakdown of carbohydrates in digestion, and keeps the soft tissues of the mouth supple, preventing sores. And saliva helps the immune system combat the invasion of numerous bacteria and viruses encountered daily. Yes, saliva intricately relates with your immunity.

Bet you did not know saliva had that many jobs!

Now that you know how important the mouth, teeth, and gums are to your health, it's up to you to decide if you want to achieve optimal oral health. Optimum oral health is the highest level of maintainable health of all the interrelated structures within and surrounding the mouth. Notice the word maintainable. Nothing, and I repeat *nothing,* is more important than having all supporting tissues of your mouth healthy *before* any restorative dental work (fillings, caps, smile makeovers, etc.) is done other than for the relief of pain or infection. Nothing.

Patch-and-repair dentistry can fix an immediate problem; for example, you break a tooth, you need a crown. But that does not return you to optimal health until you learn why the tooth broke in the first place and address that problem. A perfect mouth has good architectural patterns, stippled-like-an-orange-peel texture, perfect gum depths of less than three millimeters, excellent bone contours, and no rough edges interfering with cleaning protocol. A perfect mouth has good saliva flow and stable joints and muscles. A perfect mouth maintains health without a terrific impingement on your life habits.

You do want that, right?

So let's learn how to get on the road toward good health.

In the next chapter, I'll discuss cavities, gum disease, and one of the most overlooked aspects of good dental health, the jaw.

"Health and disease don't just happen to us. They are active processes issuing from inner harmony or disharmony, profoundly affected by our states of consciousness, or ability or inability to flow with experience. This recognition carries with it implicit responsibility and opportunity."
MARILYN FERGUSON

CHAPTER 2

. . . .

WAGING WAR:
WHEN THINGS GO WRONG

*"The patient should be made to understand that he or
she must take charge of his own life. Don't take your
body to the doctor as if he were a repair shop."*
QUENTIN REGESTEIN

Cavities

Sun Tzu said that when one is engaged in fighting, a long time to victory dulls weapons and decreases a soldier's will. He claimed no country had ever benefited from prolonged warfare and, in order to kill the enemy, one must be roused to anger and there must be rewards for doing so. A lengthy campaign should not be the object of victory. He also said a general wins a battle by making many calculations, and Sun Tzu could see who was likely to win a battle based on how many or how few calculations had been made.

Dental professionals can easily determine which patients will succumb to dental disease because the patient did not calculate the consequences of homecare inaction. Signs of many diseases, especially dental disease, can be seen in the mouth long before a person experiences any symptoms.

This chapter discusses the three main diseases of the teeth: cavities, periodontal (gum) disease, and occlusal (bite) disease. Once you know the disease process, you can calculate the necessary provisions to attack them without a lengthy campaign.

Because the American Dental Association has had a dental education campaign in place since the early 1950s, cavities constitute the most well-known tooth disease. Cavities occur when the protection of the enamel breaks down and bacteria enter the dentin. A hole forms in the tooth, allowing more bacteria to enter even deeper into the dentin. But if enamel is the hardest known living substance, how does a hole form in it?

A very thin film of saliva, known as the pellicle, covers and protects the enamel from the acids forming in the mouth due to food particles remaining on or around the teeth. If the pellicle remains undisturbed—you do not remove it daily with a toothbrush and dental floss—it thickens from the amount of bacteria growing within and becomes known as plaque. Putting it simply, plaque plus acid equals cavities. So if saliva neutralizes acids caused by fermenting bacteria, where does the acid come from?

To understand the role of saliva, let's take a quick look at nutrition.

Carbohydrates are nothing more than a long chain of simple sugars connected in various ways, forming different types of energy-producing nutrients. Carbohydrates come in numerous forms; the most familiar are the dry carbohydrates, like bread, crackers, biscuits, cakes, and pastries. Ptyalin, a saliva enzyme, transforms starchy carbohydrates into simple sugars for easy digestion. (Chewing bread long enough makes it taste sweet because of ptyalin.) These salivary juices are acidic.

All the grooves on the molar tables and all the spaces under the gums and between the teeth form excellent hiding places for bacteria, or plaque. When you do not brush properly or floss this plaque layer off the teeth, the bacteria continue fermenting, overriding the pellicle protection. Now you have the acid from the fermenting bacteria—plaque—and the additional acids from the breakdown of carbohydrates—sugar—leaving the enamel vulnerable and no longer protected from destruction.

Other acids, such as those from soda pop, work exactly the same way. But as beverages, the acids tend to sit on top of the gumline, fermenting the bacterial plaque there instead of on the biting tables.

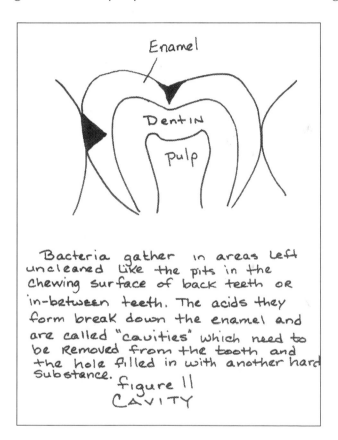

Enamel

Dentin

Pulp

Bacteria gather in areas left uncleaned like the pits in the chewing surface of back teeth or in-between teeth. The acids they form break down the enamel and are called "cavities" which need to be removed from the tooth and the hole filled in with another hard substance. figure 11
CAVITY

Cavities do not form overnight. They occur in several stages, allowing you time to prevent destruction. Acid on enamel opens the "pores" of the enamel, making it appear a cloudy white color. This white patch marks the first sign of tooth destruction, which becomes a cavity. Catching the white spot at this stage becomes critical, as the enamel ions can be reversed back to strong, solid enamel. Diligent home care and fluoride ions must be applied, but the enamel will recrystallize if the bacteria-laden plaque is thoroughly removed. Left alone, however, the white spot darkens to a brownish color as the chemicals from food and beverages continue eating the enamel. Eventually, they break through the enamel into the underlying dentin. Once bacteria breaks through, you have a cavity. The bacteria must be cleaned out thoroughly, and some type of filling material must be used to rebuild and seal the hole.

So, plaque plus acid equals cavities. No plaque, no cavity. Acid can still erode the enamel, but a cavity will not form if you diligently remove the plaque daily. Cavities are 100 percent preventable, regardless of your genetics. Make the calculations specific to your habits and assure victory over cavities.

Gum Disease

According to the Centers for Disease Control and the American Dental Association, some form of gum disease affects 80 percent of the US population. Gum disease occurs when plaque settles under the gumline space between where you see the gum and where it attaches to the tooth.

Let's compare your gums to your fingernails. Look at the top of your fingernail and then where the nail attaches to the finger bed, the quick. This can be any length from one millimeter to several millimeters. If you dig in the garden, dirt accumulates under the fingernail. Short fingernails, those two or three millimeters long, clean easily with soap and water. Maybe a fingernail brush may be needed, but the result is quickly achieved.

Longer fingernails, on the other hand, need much more thorough detailing to come clean. Nails longer than four or five millimeters (about a quarter-inch) need a nail brush to get cleaned. Different angles of the brush must be used, along with the scraping action of an orangewood stick to get out the dirt that settled at the quick. Then, another scrubbing with the brush, another look-over, and possibly another scraping and brushing may still be needed to fully clean the dirt from your nails.

The gumline makeup is exactly the same. The space where you see the gum and the part that attaches to the tooth is a pocket-like formation that collects plaque, which is laden with bacteria. The bacteria feed off the blood supply of the gums. When that runs low, they attack the bone for the nutrients they need to survive. A vicious cycle forms when the plaque remains under the gumline for any period of time. The plaque mineralizes after twenty-four hours to a rock-hard substance called tartar (dental professionals call it calculus). Being hard and rough, the tartar now accumulates plaque more readily. Bacteria cling to the hard surface quickly and do not brush off as easily any more.

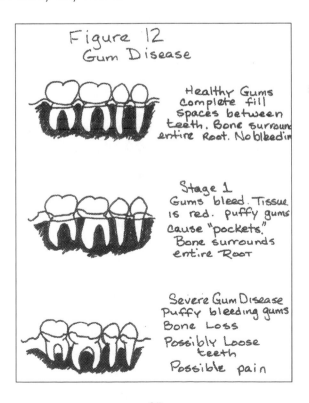

Figure 12
Gum Disease

Healthy Gums
Complete fill
Spaces between
teeth. Bone surround
entire Root. No bleedin

Stage 1
Gums bleed. Tissue
is red. puffy gums
Cause "pockets."
Bone surrounds
entire Root

Severe Gum Disease
Puffy bleeding gums
Bone Loss
Possibly Loose
teeth
Possible pain

Plaque mineralizes into tartar when left undisturbed for twenty-four hours. In smokers, it can mineralize in six hours. Tartar left under the gumline causes the bacteria to eat away at the tooth-supporting bone to get the nutrients they need to survive. You do not want them to survive. You need to get that toothbrush angled to remove the plaque daily. Like your fingernails after working in the garden, "dirt" sits under your gums. The difference is, however, how often do you work in the garden? How well do you wash your hands afterward?

How often do you put food or anything in your mouth? How often do you wash your teeth after... catch the drift here?

Once tartar forms, a hygienist must get her sharp instruments down under the gumline to disrupt and remove the colonized bacteria living there. Until this procedure is complete and all bacterial colonies are removed, you remain in a vicious cycle of unhealthy gums. Bone lost to disease does not grow back. Ever.

If you fall and break your arm, proper repositioning of the bone and casting a splint over the arm so the bones do not move while healing allowing them to heal well and strong. Gangrene in your foot, however, where the infection spreads into the bone, cannot be reversed, and your foot must be amputated. Periodontal disease attacks bone similarly to gangrene. Irreversible damage. The teeth must be "amputated," or taken out.

The first sign of periodontal disease, bleeding gums, is a huge warning to you that your gums are unhealthy. Just as your scalp does not bleed when the shampoo girl scrubs it clean—and you'd freak out if it did—neither should your gums bleed even when the hygienist scrapes them clean. Healthy gums do not bleed. If your gums bleed when you brush or floss, or while getting a cleaning at your dental office, that should alert you to stop an unhealthy process. It's no different than freaking out if your scalp bleeds at the hair salon.

Bleeding gums, otherwise known as gingivitis, is reversible, and if you keep the plaque off and out from under the gumline, you prevent periodontal disease from invading your body. To say your gums "have always bled" acknowledges that you've never taken the time to properly remove the plaque and bacteria from under the gumline.

One more analogy: Take out your spring jacket and pull the pockets inside out. Spring jackets generally have small pockets to put your keys into. How much lint sits in the bottom of the pockets? Maybe a little bit, but most likely none.

Now take out your winter parka. Parkas have deep pockets to keep your mittens in as well as your hands, your keys, and other necessities for winter warmth. Pull the pockets inside out. Notice how much lint was stored in your parka pockets over the season. And you thought you cleaned it before storing it away for the summer! It's not easy cleaning out deep pockets, is it?

Now, can you understand why your gums "have always" bled in the past? Deep pockets of gum tissue need deeper cleaning requirements and techniques to remove all the damaged "lint" stuck down there. Bleeding is the body's way of informing you that something is wrong, whether it be a bloodshot eye, blood in your stool, cat-scratched arms, a bleeding ulcer, or bleeding gums.

No plaque, no periodontal disease. Periodontal disease is 100 percent preventable in most cases.

One of the cases making it difficult to treat gum disease is occlusal disease. Occlusal disease is when the biting connection between the teeth does not properly match because of jaw dysfunction, missing teeth, misaligned teeth, fillings that are too large, or habits such as clenching or grinding teeth.

When a tooth hits with an unnatural force or against the natural plane of forces, the tooth moves. This movement stretches and pulls those nerve fibers holding the tooth in the socket. Bacteria find a new haven to settle into. Now you battle two enemies simultaneously: the force of the combative bite and the dangerous loitering bacteria. All the scraping in the world by a hygienist cannot heal this wound until the trauma is removed.

The reverse of this can also happen. Gum disease causes bone loss, creating mobility in the tooth socket. Now the tooth moves to a different position, and the bite offsets to accommodate. As long as the tooth remains mobile, the diseases continue and the teeth continue to move. As long as the bacteria linger within, the diseases continue and bone loss progresses.

Loose teeth can be managed by removing causative factors, such as correcting the interference in the bite or by splinting the teeth into their proper alignment. However, once mobility happens with teeth, the prognosis is bad, even though numerous therapies can delay the inevitable outcome.

Jaw Disease

Sun Tzu said that a general listening to counsel and acting upon it will conquer and be retained in command, but one not listening would find defeat and dismissal. In listening to the counsel, however, you need to avail yourself of any helpful circumstances beyond the ordinary and modify your plans as needed.

Circumstances beyond the ordinary in dental health mean paying attention to how the jaw functions and noting any deviations from normal based on the symptoms the patient gives the doctor, or the signs the doctor notices. By listening to and acting on the observed signs and symptoms, the jaw can regain health leading to an overall win.

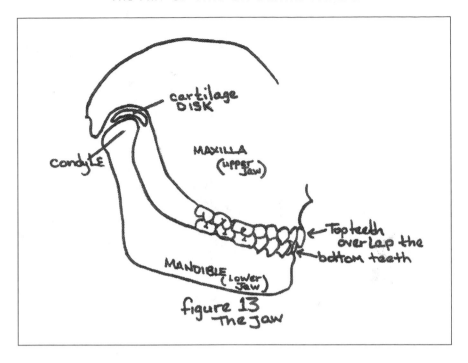

cartilage DISK

MAXILLA (upper jaw)

condyle

←Top teeth over lap the bottom teeth

MANDIBLE (lower jaw)

figure 13 The jaw

The temporal skull bone and the mandibular jawbone comprise one of the most complex joints of the body, called the temporomandibular joint or TMJ. More people have become aware of this joint lately, as TMJ has become a hot topic in the health community. Diseased or injured TMJs are called TMD, TMJD, or temporomandibular joint dysfunction. (To say you have TMJ is the same as saying you have an elbow, knee, or ankle.)

The jaw joint is the most complex joint in the body. Dozens of muscles within the face, skull, and neck work together to allow your jaw to move for speech, expressions, and chewing.

The maxilla—your top jaw—is fixed within the skull. It does not move. The top housing of the jaw joint where the socket is also remains fixed to the skull in the temporal bone, so it does not move, either.

The mandible—your lower jaw—moves. The only thing connecting it to the skull is muscles, tendons, and ligaments. The very top ball of the jawbone, the condyle, fits into the socket of the temporal bone (with a lubricating cartilage disc separating them) and determines where the lower teeth close up into the top teeth.

The TMJ functions in two ways. First, it acts as a hinge axis, like opening and closing a door, which is the function most often used for the jaw in normal talking and chewing. Second is translation action, which is when the jaw slides forward and down to open the mouth wide, like when you have to yell at the kids or bite into a polish sausage sandwich.

Translation action is similar to trying to push a rock over the top of a hill—that feeling just before reaching the top point of the hill, just as the rock is tipping over the top of the cliff. A cartilage disc separates the two bones for ease in gliding the joint open and closed. Translation is where the lubrication from the disc helps most, as the condyle glides over the sulcular cliff.

The jaw represents the only joints in the body whose right and left sides move simultaneously—one bone, two joints. No other bone crosses the middle of the body as one bone. You have two hips, a right and a left. When you need a hip replacement, the doctors first do one side then the other side. You can move one hip and not the other, like hula dancers do. You cannot do this with your jaw. When you move the right side, the left side moves also.

Jaw pain or complications can be caused by many different things, making it difficult to diagnose. Telling your dentist you have jaw pain is like telling your cardiologist you have chest pain. Chest pain can be anything: a pulled rib muscle, a broken rib, an ulcer, heartburn, acid reflux or GERD, an upset stomach, or even a heart attack.

Jaw pain can be anything, too: a toothache, sinus infection, ear infection, pulled muscle or muscle spasm, nerve impingement, artery damage, whiplash, or even a deranged disc in the joint.

The muscles used to work the jaw joint, allowing it to open and close as well as move side-to-side for chewing, speech, or expressions, are some of the strongest muscles in the body, especially for their size. Chewing a raw piece of meat or carrot or breaking open a nut requires great strength, yet this joint allows the function without much trouble.

Numerous muscles work together to open the mouth in hinge (normal talking and chewing) activity; more join in for translation. Several other muscles work together to close the mouth, which when in full contraction—closed—produce pressures equivalent to 300 pounds per square inch. Even with all this pressure, these muscles, along with the billions of nerves holding the teeth within their sockets, prohibit the teeth from contacting each other unless you consciously or subconsciously put them together, as in clenching or grinding, which can be so strong that migraine headaches can result.

Every time your doctor analyzes the bite, she must start by analyzing the jaw joint. If disharmony exists, there will be dysfunction that can show up as joint pain, muscle pain, tooth pain, or tooth mobility. All dentistry must start in the joint. Fixing a broken tooth without first analyzing why the tooth broke, or determining if there is a bite discrepancy, will lead to more teeth breaking or joint problems in the future. You can get the broken tooth fixed, but you must eventually get the bite analyzed or more teeth will eventually break. That is, of course, provided you were not chewing frozen Milk Duds, which caused the tooth to break.

Every personal anatomy differs in this regard. No one TMJ pattern fits any two people. Your particular jaw and skull anatomy, combined with your particular tooth arrangement, combined with your particular habits, determines your TMJ health.

Complicating matters more, if the jaw falls out of alignment, numerous other problems can result, such as neck or back pain, toothaches, migraine headaches, or breaking teeth due to the muscle pull.

Diagnosing problems with the jaw requires a plethora of observations on how the jaw, jaw muscles, and teeth intermingle with each other. Here are a few of the things a doctor examines:

- The musculature—-do the opening and closing muscles work in conjunction with each other like the biceps and triceps do?
- Do the muscles have any tenderness when touched (palpated)? When someone squeezes your bicep, you feel the squeeze, but you do not have pain. The jaw muscles should respond with that same sensation exactly.
- How easily does the jaw open from hinge position to translation?
- How wide can the jaw open?
- How far to the left and then to the right can the jaw easily slide over?
- How much noise happens in the jaw joint during movement, and during what movements does it occur—-open, close, hinge, translation, or all of the above?
- Does the jaw lock at any time? Where or when?
- When closing the jaw into proper centric relation, do the muscles fight the position?
- When closing into proper centric relation, does any tooth hit first before all other teeth? Which one? How much does the jaw slide after that hit before all other teeth touch?
- Do any teeth show any signs of wear facets from grinding?

- Do any back teeth touch during side to side movements or do the canines properly keep the back teeth from touching?
- Do the canines or incisors show any wear patterns? Where?
- Do any teeth have any movement during biting? What is the periodontal condition of those teeth? If no gum disease is present, why does the tooth move?
- Do any of the teeth have divots present at the gumline, indicative of clenching or hard toothbrushing?
- Does the patient complain of any pain, noise, concerns, or knowledge of clenching or grinding?
- What is the bite classification?
- What is the jaw classification?
- Do any teeth show any cracks or craze lines?

All of these questions need answers before even one filling is placed in your mouth, especially if the doctor notices any of these signs during a routine observation. But you can see the tediousness involved. Doing the complete bite analysis—for many reasons, some yours, some the doctor's—is not always possible.

One patient who agreed to this complete analysis and treatment told me, one year after completion, that he never knew how little he chewed his food before and how he felt so much better now that he could chew. However, I've also had many others who have said things like, "I'm never gonna change, so why bother paying all that money?"

Chewing food should not change the anatomy of teeth. Flattened and worn edges on the incisors or occlusal tables indicate excess muscle forces causing shearing action on the enamel. Divots in the sides of the tooth indicate excess compressive forces on the tooth. Diagnostics are tedious for both the doctor and for you. But when the doctor sees the signs and calls them to your attention, you know you have a problem. Ignoring it does not make it go away. When you find a lump in your body somewhere, even if you have no pain, you still see a doctor for diagnosis and treatment. Do the same for your teeth.

When you hit a back tooth during side-to-side jaw movements, either in chewing or by having a grinding habit, you bruise the fibers connecting the tooth to the socket. You have pain, and you want immediate relief.

The problem becomes difficult if the diagnosis does not include a bite analysis. A root canal fixes the pain, but not the problem, and eventually the tooth breaks or the pain returns afterward because the nerve to the tooth didn't cause the pain. The nerve fibers connecting it to the socket did. Those nerves remain untouched in root canal therapy.

Treating this type of problem can be as simple as grinding off the part of the tooth touching during the side-to-side movement, a process called equilibration—sort of like filing your finger nails. Yes, once that part of the tooth is filed down, it never comes back, so this is an irreversible treatment. However, when properly diagnosed and treated, it permanently saves the tooth without needing a root canal or any kind of filling, as the enamel remains intact, if caught early enough.

Many times the patient has huge amalgam or composite fillings that have weakened the enamel instead of opting for a type of filling that can protect the enamel, such as an onlay or crown. An onlay lies on top of the chewing surface to protect the weakened cusps from breaking. A crown covers the entire enamel part of the tooth, protecting it like a thimble over your finger protects the fingertip while sewing.

If the bite is good, the tooth remains okay with the large filling. Sometimes the bite remains good several years, then one day, *pop!*

There goes the tooth. True, it had a large filling and was vulnerable, but why now?

You hit it with the wrong biting forces, plain and simple. Probably you sensed the bite changed, either with this filling that you "got used to" or another filling later that "never felt quite right." Or you started a bad habit, like grinding.

Your teeth, because of those millions of nerve fibers, can feel the presence of a single hair between them. You know when the bite changes, but because of self-preservation, the mouth muscles adapt to avoid this monstrosity and you "get used to it." But your brain never does. The bite has been altered, and you have occlusal disease.

Many times, during an examination the hygienist or the doctor tells you a tooth needs a crown or onlay. Most times you say okay, and that's that. Then, several months or even a couple of years later, you return with a broken tooth, sheepishly admitted as "the one you told me about."

Another seemingly unrelated problem related to jaw misalignment is balance. The mandible consists of a thick, large, dense bone. When at rest, the lips close, but the teeth do not touch. The jaw rests in place and is held by the closing muscles.

When you stand still and look directly up, like standing under a tall tree and looking up to the top of it, your lips separate, allowing the jaw to drop slightly to maintain balance so you don't topple over backwards. In conjunction with your big toes digging into the ground, the jaw stabilizes us upright as bipeds. Similarly, when the jaw changes or becomes out of alignment, posture changes.

Mouth breathers keep their lips separated, causing the jaw to hang lower than necessary at rest. Eventually this weight pulls the skull forward and down. Human eyes are designed to see level to the horizon. When your head tilts down due to the weight of the jaw, this forces the eyes to see aslant to the horizon; hence, you subconsciously tilt your head upward to see level. Over time, the force of gravity causes bending of the spine, leading to the formation of a humpback.

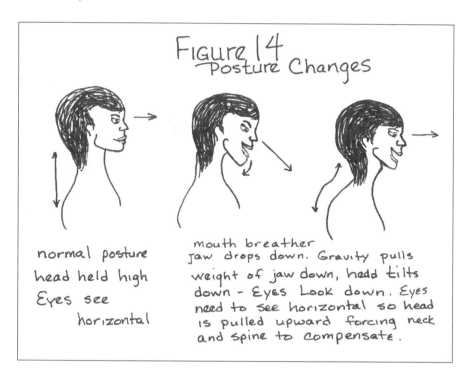

FiGure 14
Posture Changes

normal posture
head held high
Eyes see
horizontal

mouth breather
jaw drops down. Gravity pulls weight of jaw down, head tilts down - Eyes Look down. Eyes need to see horizontal so head is pulled upward forcing neck and spine to compensate.

Diagnosis of jaw disease, TMJD, is not as easy or as quick as diagnosing cavities or gum disease. The most difficult part comes from the day-in, day-out exams and treatments with no pain or obvious risk factors like in cavities or gum disease. Also, patients without pain generally neglect to follow up with treatment as recommended.

Looking at the diagnostic questions I listed, diagnosing occlusal disease can be tedious for both you and the doctor. Many boundaries exist, especially with the patient, who may have financial concerns, time constraints, emotional issues, mental concerns, or physical problems.

Some boundaries reside with the doctor, such as time constraints, skill level of the doctor or staff or lab technicians, or the availability of specialists to coordinate schedules.

Many times the patient may be aware of the problem and expect perfect results because they had treatment done. The human body, let alone human skills, cannot always guarantee perfect results, and unrealistic expectations prohibit good results from happening. Restrictions and boundaries interfere with perfect results. But eliminating or at least alleviating pain allows moving forward toward optimal health and prevents the otherwise inevitable death of the teeth.

When your dentist informs you that he sees signs of occlusal disease, listen to his or her counsel and act upon it so as not to suffer defeat.

Summary

Cavities form when plaque mixes with acid to destroy enamel. No plaque, no cavities. Gum disease occurs when plaque sits in the gum sulcus—the pocket—too long and the bacteria feed off the blood supply of the gums and supporting bone. No plaque, no gum disease.

The common denominator is plaque. Get rid of the daily plaque buildup, and you prevent these two diseases. In preventing these two diseases of the teeth, you prevent the need for dental repair treatment, which decreases the risk of getting occlusal disease.

Sun Tzu told us that to kill the enemy, one must be roused to anger and then must be rewarded upon defeating them. Let your great object be victory and not a lengthy campaign.

So, are you angry now? Are you ready to declare war on plaque? Are you prepared to receive the reward of good health and strong teeth that last in your mouth your entire lifetime? Are you ready to consider going through proper diagnostics to achieve predictable results?

Then continue reading to learn to develop strategies that defeat plaque every time. Get back to health and keep it that way!

March on, soldier!

*"I swear, if Colgate comes out with one more type of toothpaste…
I just want clean teeth, that's all I want. I don't want the tartar
and I don't want the cavities. And I want white teeth. How
come I have to choose? And then they have the 'Colgate Total'
that supposedly has everything in there. I don't believe that for
one second. If it's all in the one, how come they make all the
others? Who's going, "I don't mind the tartar so much..?"*
ELLEN DEGENERES

CHAPTER 3

· · · · · · · · · · · · · · · · · · · ·

STRATEGY

"I brush my teeth with a Sonicare toothbrush before every show."
DAVID COPPERFIELD

Proper Toothbrushing

Sun Tzu begins his chapter on strategy by saying that the best thing is to take the enemy country whole and intact. If you fight and conquer but only by destroying, you're not excellent in what you do. Supreme excellence comes from breaking the enemy's resistance without fighting. Those millions of invisible bacteria lining your mouth are the enemy. Most of them aid your body in digestion and keeping healthy. But several of them have the ability to grow at phenomenal rates, thereby invading every part of your body should you allow them to live.

Proper toothbrushing and cleaning of the teeth and gums does not take a lot of effort, but it does need to be done correctly, or you will continue fighting a lengthy battle. Brushing your teeth like Brooke Shields does in her Colgate commercial will not get your gums clean, and it can potentially harm your gums over time. Spend some time reading this chapter; some of these tactics may feel strange, as all new things do. But proper brushing and flossing will defeat the enemy's resistance without much fight, once the technique is properly learned and implemented.

Remember the anatomy of the gums surrounding your teeth. Remember that space from where you see the gum on your tooth to where it actually attaches to the tooth, similar to your fingernails (see Figure 9). Bacteria and food find that space easily and consider it a haven, a never-ending banquet, a secure fortress. The longer you allow them to feast, the more difficult it becomes to destroy them. This is war, and you are about to take up your weapons. Your job, soldier, is to destroy their home and remove food from their table.

The first strategy is to obtain a good toothbrush. Several factors need to be considered to constitute a good toothbrush, depending on you. How well can you maneuver your hands? How well can you grasp things in your hands? How crooked or how straight are your teeth? How much gum disease—pockets deeper than three millimeters—do you have to begin with?

For a relatively straight set of teeth with healthy gums, pockets no deeper than three millimeters anywhere, and good manual dexterity and hand coordination, I recommend a straight-handle toothbrush with ultra-soft bristles. I never recommend medium or hard bristles because they cannot negotiate that space under your gum without causing some damage to this fragile tissue.

For people with several crooked teeth or tiny mouths, I recommend a smaller bristle head, like a child-size toothbrush— again, with the straight handle and ultra-soft bristles. The smaller head makes for easier maneuvering around those crevices formed where the teeth overlap.

For people with disabilities, such as arthritis of the hands, I recommend a toothbrush with a straight, but thicker handle, to allow for an easier grip. If it is difficult to find a thick enough handle to grip without pain, I recommend cutting two holes opposite each other through a tennis ball or racquetball. Then, slide the handle of the toothbrush through the ball and grip the ball. Or, place the toothbrush through the holes of a bicycle hand-grip and wrap with duct tape. Electric and sonic toothbrushes have nice, thick handles also.

Now that you have picked your toothbrush, you need to decide on toothpaste. There are hundreds to choose from, and are any wrong? Yes and no. Destroying the bacterial feast under your gums is the battle. Foam really does not matter. I often brush my teeth with no paste, and I keep my mouth meticulously clean. But there are also many reasons to use paste, so how do you decide which minty or cinnamon foam you need?

I recommend only that you find the seal of the American Dental Association on the tube or on the box it comes in. The American Dental Association has numerous criteria that must be proven before allowing the seal. If the product says it fights cavities, the company that made it has to prove a lower incidence of cavities did occur through the use of this particular product and that no other factors were involved. If the product does not have the seal, it does not mean it is not a good product—I'm only curious why the company did not bother to test for approval.

Fluoride or no fluoride? To this day, in spite of the fact that fluoride has been proven to decrease cavity formation many times over and that the amount necessary to do so has no detrimental effects, controversy remains.

Fact: fluoride ions do replace hydroxyl ions in the enamel, forming a much stronger bond so less breakdown of enamel can occur. In doing so, fluoride also causes the enamel structure to be more slippery to the attachment of bacteria. I highly recommend fluoride toothpaste for all children, all elder patients and especially those on medications that tend to cause dry mouth syndrome, and any persons suffering from highly sensitive teeth. A lethal dose of fluoride requires drinking over a thousand gallons a day of fluoridated water at one part fluoride to one million parts water, and you'd have to drink two bathtubs full daily over several months before even the mildest toxic symptoms would occur. Drinking that much water would cause water intoxication long before fluoride toxicity would come in.

Even *Consumer Reports* ("The Best of Health" June 2011), when asked about the difference between drinking tap instead of bottled water, said, "If you opt for bottled water, choose a fluoridated type."

If for any reason you have qualms about the use of fluoride, I suggest you spend a lot more time brushing your teeth to ensure no additional bacteria linger to destroy them. Fluoride ions strengthen enamel. Acid destroys enamel. Plaque causes acid formation. Remove 100 percent of all plaque daily, from the time your teeth erupt into your mouth, and you have no reason to worry about needing fluoride.

For patients suffering from gum disease, or those of you wanting a whiter smile, or patients preferring no sodium laurel sulfate or wanting all-natural products, I recommend making your own toothpaste by mixing a teaspoon of baking soda with a couple drops of hydrogen peroxide to make the baking soda pasty. This concoction has been shown to disrupt some of the latent bacteria of the mouth and has the added benefit of removing surface stains to brighten the enamel a bit.

Or you can mix the baking soda with a mashed strawberry or banana to decrease stains caused by teas or coffee. Or mix the baking soda with a few drops of mouthwash for that minty freshness. Choosing toothpaste is personal, depending on your likes, needs, and tastes.

You know which toothbrush you want, and now you have picked out your toothpaste. Place a dab of paste about the size of a pea or corn kernel onto the bristles of your toothbrush. If you personally need more, go ahead—the toothpaste companies like you using lots and lots of paste—but a kernel will do the job.

Spread the paste over each surface of your teeth, then refine your grip on the handle so it is ever so light. I recommend only using a thumb and two fingers. That's all you need for control. The bristles will fight your battle for you, not your biceps.

Place the toothbrush bristles at one end of your teeth—upper right, perhaps—and angle them right into the space where the gum and tooth meet. Think of cleaning your fingernails after a day in the garden. To get all the dirt out, you need to angle the brush into the fingernail space. The same goes for your teeth. To clean under the gums and destroy the feasting bacteria, you need to angle right at them. Use this angle regardless of the toothbrush chosen. Sonic, electric, large or small head, angle the bristles into the gum space. For manual toothbrushing, gently glide back and forth over the surfaces, feeling those bristles working into that space. Repeat several times per tooth before moving to the next section of teeth to assure total destruction. Your gums should not hurt, or bleed. How long you need to stay in each place depends on your diet and other oral habits. Soft diets (such as Mickey D's or Stouffer's because you're too tired to cook) and smoking cause bacteria to congregate more quickly and ferociously, so you need extra time per section.

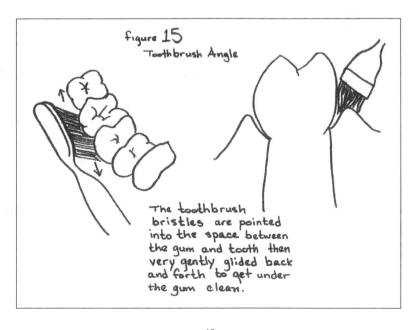

figure 15
Toothbrush Angle

The toothbrush bristles are pointed into the space between the gum and tooth then very gently glided back and forth to get under the gum clean.

When you complete the cheek surfaces of your top and bottom teeth, move to the tongue surfaces of the teeth. Because of the arch of your mouth, you need to adjust the handle of the toothbrush to reach the gumline at this angle so the bristles can destroy the bacteria lingering under that side of the teeth (see Figure 16).

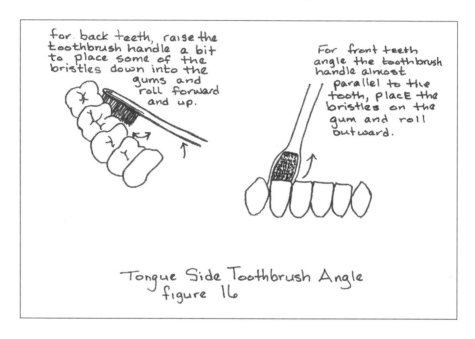

for back teeth, raise the toothbrush handle a bit to place some of the bristles down into the gums and roll forward and up.

For front teeth angle the toothbrush handle almost parallel to the tooth, place the bristles on the gum and roll outward.

Tongue Side Toothbrush Angle
figure 16

After cleaning every surface of the tongue side of your teeth well, scrub your chewing surfaces like you always have since learning to brush. Get that cookie out of there and congratulate yourself on a job well done. This entire procedure should take you about two to four minutes. Electric and sonic toothbrushes have a timer, so you can't cheat. It takes me about four to six minutes depending on the day I've had and food I've eaten to get my mouth feeling clean. Rub your tongue over every surface of your teeth and feel the smooth enamel. Any fuzzy feeling at all means you left plaque there, so go back and get that area again.

Now take several swipes with your toothbrush over the roof of your mouth and over your tongue. Yes, brush your tongue. Remember, the color of your tongue should be the same coral pink as the rest of the inside of your mouth. Go as far back to the base of your tongue as you can and brush forward. Repeat as often as necessary, rinsing frequently until all that white (or brown or black) film is removed and the coral pink color is all you see. When I use the sonic brush, I brush my top teeth for the allotted time, then my bottom teeth another round of the allotted time, then my tongue. Six minutes total with the sonic brush, as I stated above. For those of you who gag too easily and just cannot get your toothbrush to the base of your tongue, use a tongue cleaning swiper—or just take a tablespoon and proceed the same way. Go as far back as you can, swipe forward. Rinse, look, and repeat until coral pink is achieved.

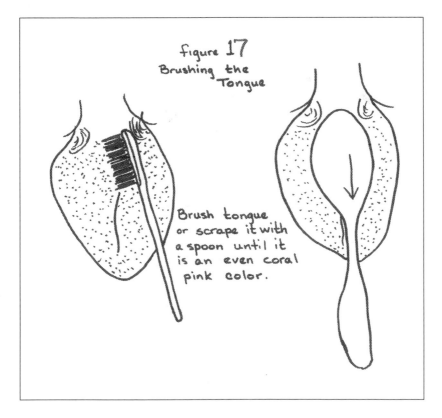

figure 17
Brushing the Tongue

Brush tongue or scrape it with a spoon until it is an even coral pink color.

Proper Flossing

I know, you all hate doing it. Okay, don't. You lose the battle hands-down. Bacteria know about this cozy haven, and they know you hate it. You want to break the enemy's resistance, so grab the floss.

String or tape floss, waxed or unwaxed, is 100 percent a personal preference. I like string, unwaxed. People with very tight tooth-to-tooth contacts may prefer waxed. People with larger spaces between teeth may prefer tape. Choose your floss and pull out a length of about eighteen inches (about forty centimeters). Using the middle finger of your dominant hand, wrap about one inch of the floss around the tip of the finger. Wrap the remaining floss around the middle finger of your other hand. This leaves the most maneuverable parts of your hand—the thumb and first finger—free to maneuver the floss.

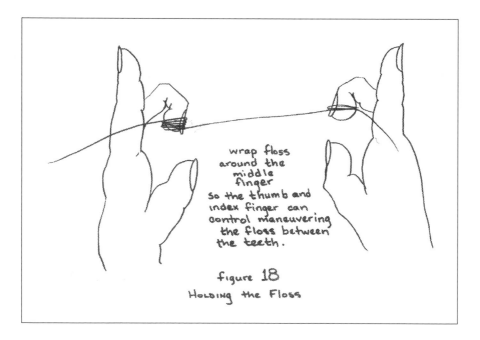

wrap floss
around the
middle
finger
So the thumb and
index finger can
control maneuvering
the floss between
the teeth.

figure 18
HOLDING the Floss

Now, between two fingers, two thumbs, or a finger and a thumb—whatever is easiest for you in each area—grasp about one inch to one and a half inches (two to four centimeters) of floss. Reach into your mouth and wrap that floss around the back end of your back tooth. Slide the floss up and down along the back surface, making sure you get under the gumline as far as it allows you to go. Imagine drying your back with a towel after a shower. Repeat up and down until the tooth feels squeaky clean, like your back feels nice and dry. This is the most often neglected area for patients who do floss. The gum behind your last tooth still comes up along that back edge. Just because no other tooth is back there, the gum still is. Clean it.

Now remove the floss from your mouth, unwrap one strand from your non-dominant to your dominate finger to get a fresh, clean piece of floss, place your hands back into your mouth, and slide the floss gently between the last two teeth. Wrap the floss backward, under the gum, and along the side of the back tooth up and down until it feels squeaky clean. Before taking this piece of floss out, bring it in front of the gum and slide the floss up and down along the back surface of the tooth in front (see illustration). Once this side of the tooth feels squeaky clean, pop the floss out from between these teeth, unwrap to another fresh area of floss, and repeat until you have made each area of each tooth surface feel squeaky clean. You can feel the squeak, so when you do not, go back in and rub into that space again. Flossing, once you master your fingers, only takes about one minute. I often floss my teeth while sitting at a red light.

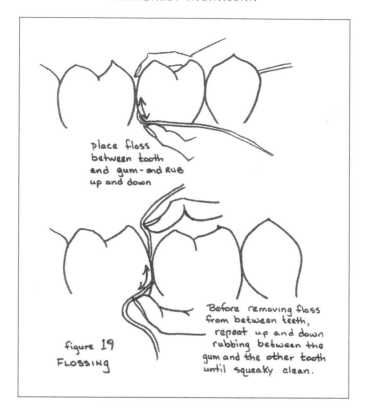

place floss
between tooth
and gum - and RUB
up and down

Before removing floss
from between teeth,
repeat up and down
rubbing between the
gum and the other tooth
until squeaky clean.

figure 19
FLOSSING

For those with dexterity problems or you who claim you just cannot get your fingers in your mouth, or if you have dental prostheses like bridges or implants, there are many flossing tools or picks to choose from, available at all drug stores. Even a water flosser (Hydrofloss™) has become available to help keep this precious area of the mouth free from bacteria. Just remember, water built the Grand Canyon, so be sure to have your hygienist or dentist teach you the proper use of this tool. The key remains the same regardless of your choice of weapon: Destroy the bacterial feast under the gumline between teeth by rubbing the tooth squeaky clean.

When camping or in third world countries, a piece of tree bark or an orangewood stick work the same way, as long as you pay attention to the angle and glide along the gumline well, removing all that fuzziness known as plaque. When you return home, resume normal toothbrushing and flossing.

Now take a swig of water or mouthwash and swish it around your mouth. Which mouthwash? Any, really. I prefer the non-alcoholic brands for most patients and the fluoridated brands for children and patients troubled by sensitivity or recurrent cavities. For my patients preferring ayurvedic care, I recommend using coconut or sesame oil. Regardless, swish hard, use those strong muscles to force the liquid between all those spaces in your mouth, including the roof, throat, and cheeks. Spend a full minute swishing. Now spit. Repeat until your mouth feels clean.

There! Less than ten minutes a day, and you achieved supreme excellence! Smokers, poor dieters, and you who are too lazy—admit it, come on—need to repeat this process more often throughout the day to thoroughly destroy the bacterial invasion, the enemy.

And now you know why your gums have always bled.

Sun Tzu says a good fighter can secure himself against defeat but can never be certain of defeating the enemy. He warns that one must take the offensive to secure against defeat and that making no mistakes can conquer an enemy who is already defeated. Take the time, be on the offensive, destroy the enemy, and get healthy!

"When it comes to eating right and exercising, there is no, "I'll start tomorrow." Tomorrow is disease.
TERRI GUILLEMETS

CHAPTER 4

· · · · · · · · · · · · · · · · · · · ·

ENERGY

"He who takes medicine and neglects to diet
properly wastes the skills of his doctors."
CHINESE PROVERB

Your Diet Affects Your Mouth

Sun Tzu maintained that direct methods of fighting (proper toothbrushing and flossing, in our case) can be used to join the battle, but indirect methods are needed to secure victory. He said that clever combatants combine direct and indirect energies, so fighting men are like a stone rolling down a steep mountainside.

In other words, food is your indirect fighting energy.

To secure victory in dental health, one needs a proper diet.

A healthy mouth needs good food. All the best brushing and flossing means nothing if your diet does not enhance the effort.

So what, exactly, constitutes a proper diet?

We learned from childhood about the four basic food groups, the food pyramid, eating a rainbow of colors, the Mediterranean diet, the high–protein and low-carb diet, blah, blah, blah. You get the point. It's not for lack of knowledge that we follow poor dietary choices. It's not even for lack of willpower. We eat poorly because we never understood the effect of combining energies to gain advantages.

I challenge you to forget about diets and think of food only as fighting energy. Just as gasoline gives a car the energy needed to get you across town to work or across the country for your vacation, good food gives our bodies the energy needed to fight bad bacteria and viruses as well as to get through the day effortlessly. You've heard it talked of as fuel for your body, because that is what it does. Food provides energy.

Some foods provide quick energy that can get you across town, if you will, but nothing more. Some provide good, strong energy, getting you clear across the country, and some foods deplete energy. Different foods employ our body defenses in so many different ways. There are foods that are good for every part of our bodies: mouth, digestion, brain, heart, and muscles. There are foods that wreak hell on our body's attempts to ward off bad bacteria and should be avoided. There are foods that are good for our overall health, but not necessarily good for our teeth. And there are all those foods in between.

Let's begin with the "bad" foods. Technically, yes, they are bad foods. Instead, think of them as foods to avoid rather than as "bad." A cold winter night curled up in front of the fireplace with a good romantic novel needs a couple of Oreos dunked in a mug of hot chocolate to complete the mood. After a long day at work, double overtime, too tired to cook anything, but starving, means a box from the freezer tossed in the microwave, right? Come on, many of you do this. Really, what's the big deal? Everything in moderation, right?

Nope. This is not healthy at all. Think more, "I know this is not a healthy choice, but I will be back on track next meal." Not tomorrow. Not next Monday. Next meal. Get back on track immediately. And if you really knew the ingredients of Oreos, well, let's just save them for that one long winter night, okay?

McFast foods, boxed foods, genetically processed foods, foods made predominately with sugar—these foods should be eaten only when absolutely nothing else is available, if at all. They provide no energy for your body. Many are nothing more than a load of chemicals joined together to taste like food. As long as customers like the taste and texture, it sells. And you're the one buying it.

But not anymore, right? If you purchase processed food, ask yourself, "processed from what?" Food grows with no need for "processing." Processed and fast "food" destroys your body; it does not energize it. Processed foods steal energy because the body has to work harder to digest the nutrients the body needs for strength and survival, if those nutrients are even available at all. Thieves! That's what they are.

When eating low-energy foods, know what havoc you wreak on your body. The bacteria in your mouth love feasting on the sugars and fight to get at it quickly, destroying your teeth. The bacteria in your gut do not know what to do with this junk and fight to figure it out. Your brain and muscles fight to find the nonexistent nourishment they need to function. Your kidneys and liver fight to rid the body of the overabundance of waste these foods create. Your colon fights to push waste out of your system. With so much fighting going on, no wonder you feel tired within a few hours after eating these foods. No wonder you do not have the energy to get through the day. Your body is at war!

When you eat these foods, know that you are putting your body through war. End the war, and get back on track quickly. Go ahead, eat the Oreos. Have the hot dog at the family barbeque. Grab that Dunkin Donuts jelly roll the boss brought in before anyone else gets it. But not every day. End the war. This battle cannot be won. Look at all that acid forming on your teeth, not to mention the fat accumulating on those hips!

Avoid these "foods" as much as possible to avoid extended battles in overall health and dental health.

Generally speaking, foods that your body needs to maintain good health also keep your teeth healthy. Raw foods like broccoli, carrots, cabbage, celery, and apples clean teeth as you chew them. By this time in life, you know the foods: apples (100 percent apple juice and natural applesauce count), apricots, avocados, bananas, berries (although some do stain your teeth, stain does not cause disease), cantaloupe and melons, cherries, grapefruit, grapes, kiwi, peaches, papayas, pears, pineapples, plums, asparagus, broccoli, cabbage, cauliflower, corn, snow peas, spinach, squash, beans, lentils, and sunflower seeds. (Whew! And that only names a few.) These foods give your body energy and also keep the mouth healthy.

Collectively we call these foods nature's toothbrush. Chew them well before swallowing, and they clean soft debris off undersurfaces of teeth, especially when eaten raw, and they clean your insides well also. Good fiber pushes everything through to eliminate the waste regularly, keeping the intestines clean and healthy and the kidneys and liver strong. Like shopping at the grocery store, your body organs find what they need, take it, and push along to the next system.

Teeth mash the food thoroughly, saliva washes it out of the mouth and down the pipes, the stomach says "aahhh" and breaks it down for the intestines that pull out all the nutrients the brain, heart, and lungs ask for. The kidneys and liver don't have much waste to eliminate, so they store what they need and gather the bulk for the colon to say, "Oh, cool, this slides out easily."

When eating nature's toothbrush foods, you never need to do a cleanse. Your body's energy systems take care of that for you. No fighting—just smooth and easy work, gathering necessities and gaining energy. Eat these foods often, and your health will stay strong, both dentally and overall. No extra acids. No extra fat.

Some foods are very healthy for the body, like whole grain breads and pastas, sweet potatoes, quinoa, oatmeal, almonds, citrus fruits, raisins, prunes, popcorn, walnuts, etc., but are not good for the teeth. The teeth have rounded edges and grooves and pits to help mash food, and the foods listed above have soft textures that easily stick in those grooves and under-surfaces of the teeth, or have acids that can erode the enamel, or small hulls that get stuck under the gum. The body needs these foods, and they should be eaten daily, but with care.

A patient who normally had great hygiene and check-ups came in one day and had six huge cavities! What changed? Well, he had decided to do a liver cleanse and began drinking lemon water every morning. I have no problem with that; I believe ayurvedic treatments work. But lemon is acid. Acid erodes enamel. Drinking the citric water would not have caused such damage, but he sipped it all morning long, like many of you do with your coffee. (And if you have those calorie-loaded lattes with sweeteners in them, you are doing the same thing to your teeth.) The acidic environment remains for twenty minutes after you swallow the food. Sipping causes the acidic lemon to remain in your mouth all morning long. Nothing washes it away, and nothing neutralizes the environment. No wonder the teeth dissolved in just a few months. (He got everything fixed up and changed his habits quickly.)

Whole grain pastas, sweet potatoes, quinoa, and the like are all carbohydrates, which begin breaking down in the mouth from the saliva. Saliva momentarily becomes more acidic as the sugars pull apart from the long chain carbohydrate.

Dried fruits concentrate all the fruit sugars for a powerful punch of energy. But saliva takes twenty minutes to wash away the remnants and neutralize again. And the stickiness of them clings to the grooves within the teeth, leaving them to sit a long time. I had a patient who thought he began eating healthy by snacking on raisins instead of chocolate candies. Another case of several new cavities in a short time alerted me to ask and learn about his dietary error. I switched him back to chocolate, but only the 80 percent dark chocolate once daily, alternating with once daily raisin snacks.

Nuts and seeds need good molars to grind them well for easier digestion and processing the fats appropriately. Some parts also stick in the teeth grooves of the molar chewing table, causing the debris to stay longer than just chewing would.

Your body needs these amazing nutrients, but your teeth can suffer from them. Like drinking instead of sipping lemon water, you need to eat these foods during meals. Combining the sticky and acidic foods with neutral and hard foods cleans the remnants off the tooth surfaces quickly, neutralizing the saliva acids more rapidly. Balancing a healthy diet assures energy for all daily activities and keeps the teeth surfaces free of debris also.

Now, what about all those foods in between, like salmon, cod, halibut, non-fat cheese, yogurt, milk, eggs, turkey, (organic) chicken, peanuts and peanut butter, etc.? They are good for you in moderate quantities, not daily. The non-sticky ones can be good for the teeth, but again, not daily. So when you do eat them, combine them with the good foods, like putting peanut butter on an apple, or having your cereal with yogurt and berries instead of milk and sugar. You may be surprised to see how good they taste and decrease the urge to have those Oreo cookies. I'm sure by now you've even heard cheese and dark chocolate actually stop cavities rather than forming them. And yes, mozzarella, cheddar, and Gouda cheeses do have calcium and other properties that inhibit bacteria by decreasing the amount of acid the saliva forms, thereby decreasing the amount of cavities that can form, and chocolate makes the enamel slippery so plaque cannot adhere so readily. But you still can't have them in large quantities and hope to never have a cavity in your life again. You'd end up hurting your body from the excess fat cheese contains.

By consciously pairing sticky or not-quite-so-healthy foods with very healthy foods, you can gain the energy needed for healthy living and keep most of the teeth surfaces clean and strong. Try reading and implementing the examples in those *Eat This, Not That* books, and substitute choices. You may even surprise yourself with wonderful new flavors!

Enjoy food. But know that what you put into your body affects all parts of health and energy. Be mindful of your choices and daily habits in eating. Eat the softer foods first, so the harder texture foods can wash the teeth afterward. Follow acidic foods with neutral foods, or rinse your mouth well with water. If choosing less healthy foods, pair them up with good, strong foods. Make your daily choices healthy ones, and when you do get off track, get back on track right away. Use food for energy, not the other way around. Caffeine beverages and sugar-filled snacks feel like they enhance your energy, but they actually deplete it. If you feel tired or have low energy, think about what foods you ate earlier in the day and recognize the direct correlation between the foods you eat and how you feel. Don't let food drain you.

Chew until all the food mashes well before swallowing it. Remember Grandma telling you to "chew all your food thirty-two times, once for each tooth"? Old-time wisdom speaks loud and clear. When you don't chew right, you can't poo right. It's all connected through one long tube.

Now, get in there and stick to your routine of good brushing and flossing. Combine your direct forces with the indirect methods, and voila! Now you have a strong, healthy, energetic body from great food choices, as well as strong, healthy teeth!

"In order to change we must be sick and tired of being sick and tired."
ANONYMOUS

"Health is not valued until sickness comes."
THOMAS FULLER

CHAPTER 5

• • • • • • • • • • • • • • • • • • •

MANEUVERING

"It is part of the cure to want to be cured."
SENECA

Mouth Diseases and Your Overall Health

Sun Tzu clearly stated that even after you assemble your army and concentrate your forces, you must blend and harmonize the different elements and do tactical maneuvering. Really tough stuff. He claimed if you send a fully equipped army out to claim an advantage, you probably already got there too late. When you maneuver an army—a single, united body—the brave cannot advance alone, and the cowardly cannot retreat alone. A united force needs to be reckoned with. An undisciplined multitude is dangerous.

The mouth and the body are one unit made up of dozens of systems. The teeth do not walk into the bathroom by themselves to brush themselves. The teeth do not walk into the dental office by themselves. Those "chatter teeth" toys are pretty cute, but no one eats with them. The teeth connect the heart to the mouth via the blood supply. The teeth connect the intestines to the mouth via the digestive process. The teeth connect the brain to the mouth via the nerves. The teeth expected to function alone retreat from the body. The body without teeth lose the war.

I mean this several ways.

First, you cannot expect good dental health if you are not caring for yourself by eating properly and getting the proper amount of rest, sleep, and exercise. Nor can you expect good overall health when your teeth and gums are uncared for and bacteria linger throughout your mouth.

The back teeth cannot chew properly and will fracture if the anterior guidance—the front teeth—break down or are missing, which impairs the jaw placement. When back teeth are missing, the design of the front teeth does not allow for proper chewing, and the teeth end up fracturing. You swallow food whole instead, resulting in digestion problems.

The body bothered by a toothache cannot function through the day.

All the elements must harmonize; all the troops must form a single disciplined unit with each performing their own unique job.

The body is one unit composed of many individual parts, each specializing in a particular craft of its own, yet depending completely on the others to complete their jobs. The mouth is one unit composed of many different types of teeth and muscles, each specializing in a particular task, yet completely dependent on each other to perform their own functions properly.

In the army you may have a scout, a sniper, a cook, a medic, and many other positions that each have a specific assignment to perform. When the scout does not get accurate information, the army can walk into an ambush. When the cook cannot feed the soldiers, they have no energy with which to fight. If a sniper cannot take out the guard, no one moves forward.

The body works exactly the same way. The heart keeps the blood moving to bring nourishment to all body parts. The lungs filter out chemicals and pour oxygen into the blood for all body parts. The liver stores all unused fats to have them ready when needed for all body parts. The kidneys clean the blood so it can return fresh to all body parts. Get the picture? The teeth chew the food so it can be digested into proper nourishment for all body parts.

Even though dentistry replaces missing teeth extremely well, food cannot be chewed properly with partial or complete dentures, or with holes where teeth used to be. Even implants, although excellent replacement parts for missing teeth, do not have the same perception in chewing because they lack those nerve fibers anchoring the tooth to bone. Digestion problems occur and overall body health diminishes whenever teeth go missing.

And it goes both ways.

Recent statistics show very high percentages of patients with gum disease are at risk for diabetes and other health problems. Also, inflammation caused by a loose tooth increases the risk of Alzheimer's disease. Gum inflammation after age seventy shows a strong association with a lower IQ than from previous testing.

Inflammation or infection in the mouth needs treatment, no differently then inflammation or infection elsewhere in the body. A wound must be cleared of the infection to heal. Oddly enough, most patients, and even some doctors, do not recognize gum disease as infection of the mouth because it progresses without pain.

So does cancer.

Nutrients in the blood supply make up salivary components. All things found in the blood are found in saliva. Saliva contains more than two thousand proteins and hundreds of different types of bacteria, with more than seven hundred species in the mouth. More than thirty of these bacteria affect the gums, and over two hundred affect the teeth.

Having bad gum bacteria living in your mouth does not mean you will get gum disease, but without these bacteria, you won't. This translates into "my teeth have always been bad" syndrome. You "always take care of" your teeth (although now you know you may not have been doing it as well as you thought), and your brother never does, and he never has cavities and you always do. You have the susceptible bacteria; he does not. Yet. (He will. You'll see.)

Antibiotics do not infiltrate the proteins covering the bacteria (plaque)—I told you bacteria love a good place to hide. A few bacteria have been found responsible for most of the disease connections and do most of the damage between body and mouth. I'll call them PG for short (*Treponema tannerelli, Tannerelli forsynthesis,* and *Porphyromonas gingivalis,* if you really wanted to learn Latin). *And* they are resistant to the body's defense system! *And* they *do invade* the blood vessel linings and the cheeks and the tongue and the tonsils! *Invade.* As in, they find their way into these areas and embed deep down into them and settle in for life. Like the proverbial mother-in-law you cannot get rid of.

A direct link has been established between PG and descending aorta aneurisms (abdominal aneurism). It is thought they may also dictate different reactions to bacteria in the gut, which end up causing diabetes, obesity, and cancer. A patient with gum disease and arteriosclerosis has a different type of arterial damage than others. Studies continue finding PG throughout the body, but only in patients with gum disease.

Gum disease (periodontal disease) is a chronic inflammatory disease of your body. Not just your gums—your whole body. An entire book can be written on this subject; that's how important it is.

No correlation has been established between the amount of plaque and the severity of gum disease. Some people get it fast and bad, and others take years for it to get bad. However, a gene has been isolated for those getting the disease prior to age twenty-five. If the gene is present, the patient needs to be considered at high disease risk and needs professional cleaning intervention every three to four months (more for smokers) to keep plaque at the utmost minimum, preventing fast and furious bone destruction.

Let's put gum disease into perspective: If you have a five-millimeter pocket on every tooth (remember that anything deeper than three millimeters you cannot clean), you have an ulcer equivalent to the size of twenty square centimeters in your gut. (That's about eight inches—quite huge! Like road rash down your entire thigh from a bicycle wipeout.) The point is, you'd pay attention to that, so why do you not pay attention to the mouth ulcer lingering under your gums?

Because the pain does not come until the disease is too far gone, like cancer.

So listen up. You are indeed hurting. PG and the others travel throughout your entire body, eating whatever they please wherever they want. Once they've checked in, they settle down and stay. Some may travel when too many occupy the same area. Like gypsies, they just want food and shelter, and they roam until they find the place to hunker down and call home within your body.

Another aspect of the mouth-body connection has been observed with some bacteria showing up in the mouth *only* if other disease is present! New research shows certain bacteria showing up in the mouth in very early stages of pancreatic and breast cancers. This can help with very early diagnostics for these diseases. Work continues on the diagnostic techniques, but our knowledge increases daily.

The difficulty in these early diagnosing techniques with a patient who has gum disease is that there are too many bacteria in the mouth that are so poorly differentiated—meaning the bacteria reproduce so rapidly, many of them never mature. Cancer cells also reproduce this rapidly. Which undifferentiated cells belong to the bacteria, and which belong to the cancer? Early detection techniques become a moot point, delaying early interceptive treatment.

Studies have found that each millimeter of bone loss due to gum disease increases the risk of tumors from the HPV virus by 2.6 times. Individuals with Crohn's disease and colitis (pretty serious intestinal disorders causing severe pain) show a significantly higher count of certain bacteria in their saliva than patients without these disorders.

The body bacteria invade the mouth, and the mouth bacteria invade the body. Treatment involves sterilization, which means all bacteria, molds, fungus, and viruses die—an impossible task in the mouth and in the entire body. In order to kill all the bacteria, we need to kill everything—*everything*. And we can't do that. Does this mean that the immune system, even with the help of antibiotics, cannot get PG under control? Pretty much, yes. Once your body becomes invaded by PG from gum disease, you have a lifelong battle disrupting and displacing colonies from here on out.

Studies continue, but we do know that by treating gum disease, CRP (creatinine reactive protein, a protein marker in your blood telling you how much inflammation your body has, thereby increasing your risk of heart attack) decreases by 18 percent. The A1C (diabetes blood sugar test) lowers by 18 percent, and blood pressure drops by 3 percent. This highly suggests gum disease as an independent risk factor in all forms of cardiovascular disease, including stroke and Alzheimer's. Gum disease affects your entire body. Considering cardiovascular disease leads the causes of death in the United States, gum disease control plays a major role in regaining heart health.

Based on the links noted between mouth health and systemic health, the mouth truly reflects the level of overall health. Many diseases show in the mouth before being noticed by the body. Examples include osteoporosis, vitamin deficiencies, protein deficiencies, adrenal problems, thyroid problems, stomach and stomach acid problems, leukemia, anemia, and numerous others. Many diseases of the body, such as diabetes and high blood pressure, intestinal and stomach problems, and even certain cancers, have an untoward effect on the mouth.

And you thought the dentist only took care of teeth.

Get your comprehensive periodontal tissue assessment annually. The exam includes the doctor checking for visual signs of inflammation (redness at the gumline instead of that uniform coral pink color), bleeding gums, loss of the gum tissue surrounding teeth (recession is *not* a normal sign of aging), loss of bone support, or any pockets deeper than four millimeters. Any of these signs present means you have gum disease. If the pockets can be controlled, the bacteria can be controlled, but remember that any pockets deeper than five millimeters are almost impossible to control. Mouthwash tends to only get one to two millimeters; toothbrushes and floss can only get two to three millimeters clean. Our instruments can get in to about five millimeters, get some tissue shrinkage by removing irritants, then reach more and repeat until the pockets stay healthy at three millimeters, or less in some cases. Others need surgery to achieve this result.

If there is no pocket reduction occurring, for your own health and wellness, see a gum specialist (periodontist) and do what it takes to get healthy. When the orthopedic surgeon tells you that you need a hip replacement, you do it. When the cardiologist tells you that you need a bypass, you do it. When your dentist tells you that you need gum treatment, do it. Your health depends on it.

The war can never be won working alone, and you gain no benefit from prolonged warfare.

"There are two things in life that a sage must preserve at every sacrifice: the coats of his stomach and the enamel of his teeth. Some evils admit of consolations, but there are no comforts for dyspepsia and the toothache."
HENRY LYTTON BULWER

CHAPTER 6

· · · · · · · · · · · · · · · · · · · ·

ATTACK BY FIRE

*"Faced with the choice of enduring a bad toothache or going
to the dentist, we generally tried to ride out the bad tooth."*
JOSEPH BARBERA

*"The man with a toothache thinks everyone
happy whose teeth are sound..."*
GEORGE BERNARD SHAW

Mouth Pain and Dental Emergencies

Sun Tzu said if it is to your advantage to make a move, do it, but if not, then stay put. He said a kingdom once destroyed can never again come into being and that the dead cannot be brought back to life. Sounds like, "Duh," but so often this advice is not followed in all aspects of life. Many of us do things without thinking and end up meeting serious consequences. Most of us have very good reasons (excuses) for not doing what should have been done.

Most of you reading this book have had dental treatment in the past, some of it not very enjoyable. Some of you have always had bleeding gums. Some of you have always had bad teeth; you got them from your mother. Don't you wish you got your father's teeth? Some of you had a dentist from hell when you were a kid and never got over it. Most of you never learned the proper way to really take care of your teeth or why that really is important to you—after all, your parents had dentures…

I could go on and on with all the excuses I've heard through the decades. And I have heard some doozies! Once I had a woman tell me she could not get the two routine check-up X-rays—bitewings— because she was hosting a dinner party later that evening. Outside of thinking maybe she didn't want a "glowing" reception, I still haven't figured that one out.

The point is you can never go back. What's done is done, and now you need to move forward. Every day, at least one patient says to me, "I'll wait till it hurts," when presented with a diagnosis needing treatment. So you wait. Then, Christmas morning, when you have absolutely no time and the doctor is out of town for the holiday, *bam!* There's your pain. You waited, you got it. Congratulations. Now what do you do?

A kingdom destroyed can never be brought back into being, and the dead cannot be brought back to life. You have pain. Something is seriously wrong. Something died or is in the process of dying.

What do you do now?

First, let's figure out what caused the pain. Remember the anatomy of a tooth. The enamel covers the outer surface, and the dentin cushions the nerve (pulp) against outside forces like speech and chewing and crushing food. The pulp likes that cushion, and whenever it decreases in size from some damage to the enamel and dentin, the pulp gets angry.

When the cavity, crack, chip, gum recession, or trauma occurs too fast, initially the pulp lays down another layer of dentin to increase the size of the cushion back to the size it likes, but eventually it cannot keep up and then rebels fiercely. Of the hundreds of nerve fibers within and surrounding the tooth, they know only one response—- pain. Whether the stimulus is heat, cold, a crack, tooth movement from trauma, gum recession, or biting your fork from eating too fast, the response is exactly the same—pain. Sometimes the pain feels dull and annoying, sometimes sharp and stabbing, but it is pain.

When the brain receives the signal that you placed ice next to the tooth, you may experience pain, but then the brain analyzes what caused the pain and sends a signal back saying, "Oh, hey, you're healthy, it's okay," and the pain stops just as quickly as it came.

But when the pain persists far too long and the nerve just finally gives up, you experience dull, achy, annoying pain that never really seems to go away. And when the trauma hits fast and furiously, the pain becomes sharp, stabbing, and unbearable. Either one may cause swelling; both need to be cared for. Now—before the swelling comes, if you haven't waited too long already. The pulp gave up and died. The dead cannot be brought back to life. You must dispose of it.

What?

To fix a tooth giving unbearable, stabbing pain or one that persists in annoying, achy pain, you must dispose of the tooth or the nerve. Root canal treatment thoroughly cleans the dead nerve tissue from the pulp of the tooth and disinfects the dentin to maintain the tooth in your mouth for you. Of course, the tooth no longer has the supporting pulp protection and becomes brittle, so you usually need to place a crown (cap) over the top so the enamel and dentin stay protected.

Should you opt out of the root canal, your option becomes extraction of the tooth. Leaving a dead pulp in your body causes the same damage as leaving dead tissue anywhere on your body. Gangrene of the toes—an infection causing the death of skin and underlying structures—when left too long causes amputation of the foot, just as death of the pulp tissue causes you to need amputation of either the nerve or the tooth entirely. The dead tissue must be removed from the body, or the body will attempt to remove it. That causes swelling, which can lead to whole body death.

What did I just say? You can die from a toothache?

Yes. Leaving the dead tooth or pulp tissue in your mouth eventually causes the "jaw" to become swollen. (It really is the soft tissues around the jaw, like the nerves and blood vessels, not the actual bones—but it feels like the entire jaw.) Not only are all these massive amounts of bacteria coursing through every blood vessel in your body, but also your entire immune system responds in high alert to put out the fire. The problem is that the fire is uncontrolled. The bacteria are winning the battle. You feel sick. Your body cannot respond. Your immune system has been weakened. If the swelling is in the upper jaw, it can get into your sinuses and eyes. If the swelling is in the lower jaw, it can block your airway. You can die.

Extracting the tooth is the fast and easy answer. (Although, do not have the tooth extracted with the swelling present unless you are in a hospital or surgeon's office because the anesthesia will not be able to get through the infection; the risk of spreading the infection further into your system increases. You need to take an antibiotic for a few days or be on an antibiotic IV, then have the extraction. So you will be in pain a few days. Severe pain, usually.) But before telling the doctor to "just pull it," think about what you just told him or her to do—remove a piece of your body. I have had patients tell me they didn't want to be bothered taking care of their teeth and asked to have them all pulled.

When you get an eye infection, do you tell your ophthalmologist to "just pull it out"? Glass eyes look real good these days. You have another eye—what's the big deal? You can't really tell the difference between the real eye and the glass eye. Still can't see out of it, though. Still have to take it out at night and clean it well, place it in a glass on the nightstand, and wash your eye socket real well before going to sleep. But they look nice.

Teeth and false teeth are no different. Dentures are a piece of plastic you shove in your mouth during the day, take out to clean your mouth after eating, and put in a glass on the nightstand before going to sleep. Altered taste buds due to the plastic encasement cause food to taste differently. Textures of food feel different. Chewing works differently—no anterior guidance. You must chew with both sides simultaneously to keep the darn thing balanced in your mouth while eating. And, like the glass eye you cannot see out of, those nerve fibers anchoring the tooth into the socket, which give you the perception of what you chew, disappeared with the extraction of the teeth. Your biting forces went from three hundred pounds per square inch down to well below one hundred. A person with full dentures can bite with all their force on my hand and not break skin or even hurt much at all, usually not even leaving an imprint on my skin.

But, okay, you had the one offending tooth pulled, and now you have a gap where a tooth used to be that you now need to replace. Remember, molars do the chewing. You put out the fire, but the ashes still smolder. Down the line, problems continue until you fix the body properly so it can function as designed. Until you remove all the smoldering ashes and rebuild, you risk more fires in the future.

Remember, in the chapter on occlusal disease and bite problems, how the jaw muscles for closing the mouth apply forces to the teeth that the tongue opposes? This keeps the teeth in the neutral zone. With the missing tooth gap, the forces have no opposition and cause shifting of all the nearby teeth (see Figure 20).

Pulling one tooth instead of caring for it with a root canal or replacing it properly causes an entire forest fire. Yes, the pain went away, but the ashes remain smoldering as the teeth continue shifting. The mouth now tries working with an unbalanced bite, which causes stress from the chewing interferences, which causes stress on the jaw joints, which causes more unwanted movements during chewing, which causes more digestion issues… sigh. This cycle endures over the course of years or even decades. The damage continues until you replace the missing body part.

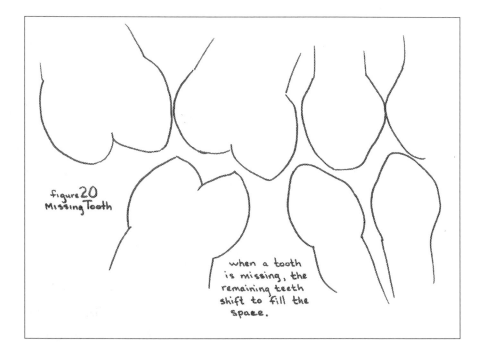

figure 20
Missing Tooth

when a tooth is missing, the remaining teeth shift to fill the space.

Root canals remove all the dead tissue and disinfect the affected dentin. The doctor opens the dentin to access the pulp and removes all the dead and infected nerve tissue from the tooth. Disinfecting cleansers wash the dentin well, and a natural rubber-based material called gutta percha fills the gap where the nerve used to be and seals the hole from recurring bacteria that may linger, seeking new homes. With the fire now gutted and extinguished, rebuilding begins, and a crown fits over the outside structures of the tooth to protect it from further damage. Just as a thimble fits over your finger to protect it from being pierced by a needle while sewing, the crown protects the tooth from forces to the brittle substructure that no longer receives nutrients from the body.

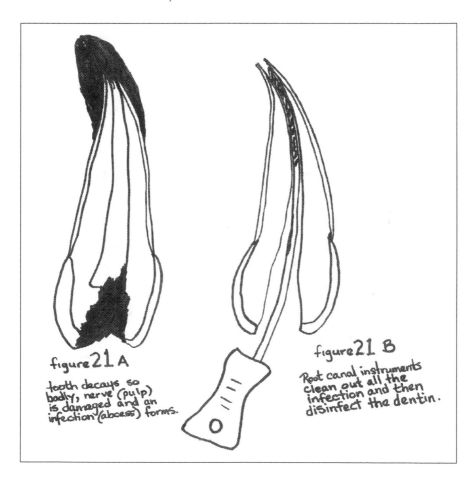

figure 21 A

tooth decays so badly, nerve (pulp) is damaged and an infection (abcess) forms.

figure 21 B

Root canal instruments clean out all the infection and then disinfect the dentin.

I just talked about the biggest fire—a tooth infection, which can lead to a shifting bite from tooth loss, which leads to injuring your entire bite. The bite change eventually causes other health problems, such as migraines, lower back pain, TMJD, and poor digestion. The muscles must compensate for the changed bite, and chewing forces decrease. The entire health system is altered.

Many other types of fires exist. If you put bread in the toaster and it gets stuck and stays in so long it catches fire, you can easily put this fire out by unplugging the toaster, removing the bread (well, burnt toast), and smothering the fire with a dishtowel. Pull out the stuck toast, clean the toaster, plug it back in, and you're good to go. Similar small fires happen in the mouth, as well.

Popcorn: one healthy food I do not eat. Many patients (actually, I average about one patient every other week with this complaint) have a sore and swollen gum around a tooth they need checked. Sure enough, I retrieve a popcorn hull stuck under the gum, and they last ate popcorn three or four days earlier. Like a sliver in your finger, a popcorn hull under your gum hurts. A fire, but a small one.

Upon removing the popcorn hull, the gum reverts back to normal within hours. Your dentist uses a small bit of anesthetic (novocaine is the generic name you may know) and scrapes under the gum down into the pocket—remember, you are otherwise healthy and the pocket is only two to three millimeters—and the offending problem comes out. You go home and feel great by morning.

If your dental health has slackened and your pocket depth sits at the four- or five-millimeter range, getting food debris stuck under the gum can resort to a medium-level fire. More pain. More damage. More difficult to extinguish. A medium-level fire can be irreversible, like the wildfire of an abcess, or only a bit more damaging than the popcorn.

Chewing frozen Milk Duds (yes, people do this) can break a tooth in half, causing the pulp to scream. Often a sedative ointment (like clove oil–based medicaments) calms everything down until we rebuild the cracked tooth properly.

Grinding or clenching teeth causes shearing stress forces on the enamel, leading to cracked teeth. Many times a cusp pops off a bicuspid or molar, but no pain occurs because the pulp still maintains a good dentin cushion. Here, treatment can wait until the reason the tooth broke in the first place can be assessed. Remember, teeth survive airplane crashes. The tooth did not break by itself. Something caused it. Eliminating the reason for the break needs to occur first, then the rebuilding of the tooth. If you only crown the tooth without finding the reason for the break in the first place, other teeth will break in the future.

Sometimes, depending on the severity of the break, a root canal may be the best option to prevent future breakages of that tooth (see Figure 21B). Building a strong foundation under the gum helps protect the weakened core structure above the gum, and then placing a crown over the top strongly binds everything together.

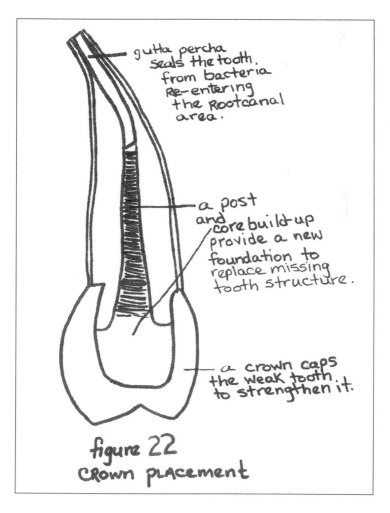

gutta percha seals the tooth from bacteria Re-entering the Rootcanal area.

a post and core build-up provide a new foundation to replace missing tooth structure.

a crown caps the weak tooth to strengthen it.

figure 22
Crown placement

Trench mouth is another medium fire encountered often. Sounds gross, and it is. The proper name we call it is ANUG—-acute necrotizing ulcerated gingivitis. **Necrotizing** means tissue is dying. **Ulcerated** means it's an open-sore wound. **Acute** means it came on suddenly. **Gingivitis** means inflammation of the gums. So this disease is an ulcerated, dying gum infection. Of course, the disease did not occur suddenly, but the pain seems to come from out of nowhere.

Plaque overrides the gum tissues so severely in ANUG that the bacteria eat away at the gums, hence the ulcers. The cause generally links to stress in addition to the excessive plaque buildup. First diagnosed during the Great War on the soldiers fighting in the trenches—severe stress and no way to brush and floss—gave it its name.

Treatment feels almost as painful as the disease, even with anesthetic, but removing the plaque begins the healing process rapidly. Relief comes instantly, but the gum damage remains for life.

Viruses infiltrate the mouth as easily as they infect any part of the body. HPV—human papillomavirus, more commonly known as genital warts—occurs in the mouth, as can genital herpes. Yes, genital infections occur in the mouth. The mouth often plays an active role in lovemaking. If the virus can occur in the genitals, it can get in the mouth when the mouth visits the area. Treatment for the mouth or the genital area uses the same medications.

The same with yeast infections—candidiasis. Although yeast grows anywhere warm and moist when immunity becomes compromised for any reason, when it occurs in the mouth (yes, guys, you can get it too) we usually need to treat the entire digestive tract. Treatment for yeast infections can be long and tedious and sometimes never fully resolved, depending on your immune system, how long it invaded you, and how well you follow directions in therapy.

Severe gum disease, where teeth move and you actually have pain, can be one of the most severe mouth diseases affecting the body. Waiting until it hurts or bothers you causes the inflammation to rapidly become infection because of the bacteria lingering under the gum ligaments down into those nerve fibers anchoring the tooth to bone. This leads to the tooth moving in the socket, which leads to more bacteria entering the pocket and your blood stream, which can now spread to other teeth and body parts, which can mean several or all teeth need to be pulled to prevent further spread of infection throughout the entire body. Wow! Even if the pain is minimal, like only when you chew something hard and the tooth moves, the disease and bacteria continue spreading. They want a happy home with a big feast, and when the neighborhood gets crowded, many pack up and move. Putting out this fire entails a very long process.

Saliva: once again the forgotten entity of the mouth. Lack of or decrease in saliva flow causes severe cavities, mouth sores, immunity problems, digestion problems, swallowing problems, and burning tongue or lips syndrome. Do not underestimate the role of saliva. Over one hundred medications decrease salivary flow. Blood pressure medications, diabetes medications, and ulcer medications, to name a few, cause severe dryness of the mouth, which can cause not only disease issues, but also pain. Mouth sores run rampant when no saliva can wash bacteria away.

Treating mouth sores becomes very difficult when there is no moisture to alleviate the pain. When the patient tries to treat it themselves, only making matters worse, like putting an aspirin directly on an aching tooth. Aspirin is an acid. Acid burns. Now you have a toothache, which cannot be treated until after the burn heals. This has happened so often, I wonder if people tape aspirin to their foreheads to alleviate a headache. Do not make a fire on top of an existing fire.

The best treatment for all dental emergencies is to never have an emergency in the first place. Of course, car accidents or getting hit in the mouth with a racquetball racquet (Where was your mouth guard?) can never be predicted, but most "fires" can be prevented with proper care of the teeth, gums, and mouth, and with good overall health in general. Good toothbrushing and flossing, regular exams so trained eyes can see what you do not see, a healthy diet, proper rest, and exercise keep strength and energy alive, and as a result, your teeth and body stay vivaciously alive as well. If you keep your mouth and body prepared and healthy, the only fires will be accidents.

Fires occurring in an otherwise healthy mouth—such as heavily bleeding gums and absolutely no plaque or tartar anywhere at all—should cue your dentist or physician to look at other systems of the body, such as diabetes, leukemia, pancreas problems, lack of nutrients or vitamin deficiencies, or other problems that can show up orally before the symptoms show bodily.

Leaving the lights on with a Christmas tree not sitting in a water pot can start your house on fire. Or an outdoor tree can be hit with lightning, starting a fire. Both cause fire to the tree, but one accidentally happened—the other you intentionally caused. Okay, unintentionally, perhaps, but you caused it. You neglected to keep the water pot full.

Accidents happen, but don't sit and wait for them or cause them unintentionally. Take action when it is to your advantage to do so. When the doctor diagnoses a problem, fix it so you never have to worry about destruction to your kingdom.

CHAPTER 7

. . . .

THE USE OF SPIES

*"No, my friend, I am not drunk. I have just been to the
dentist and need not return for another six months!
Is it not the most beautiful thought?" Poirot*
AGATHA CHRISTIE: <u>ONE TWO BUCKLE MY SHOE</u>

Choosing Your Health Care Providers

Sun Tzu talked a lot about spies. When you march a thousand men great distances, you entail a heavy loss on the people and heavy drain on resources. One begrudging the spending of silver is no leader at all and cannot achieve victory. Having foreknowledge enables a good general to strike, conquer, and achieve things beyond the ordinary man. A wise general uses the highest intelligence for spying to achieve great results. An army depends on spies, just as a body depends on other eyes watching for signs things may be abnormal.

You are the general of your army fighting against poor dental health. Who are you going to employ as spies? How do you know if they are doomed spies or surviving spies? Good spies or bad spies? How do you choose a health care provider who helps you in victory or one that endangers your outcome? How do you know when the spending of silver (paying the fees) is fair and just, or too much? How do you validate new carpet, a trip to Hawaii, and a Bahamas cruise, yet have no money to pay those dental fees? Are you prepared to take the heavy drain on your system, especially now that your awareness of the overall health effect happening to you? Be the wise general and use your spies.

These questions take a lot of things into consideration. No one can make the choice on trusting your spies but you. Trust the wrong ones, and the war is over. You lost. Dentures, or worse. Some mouths or some people just cannot wear dentures. No teeth to chew food with means no good healthy food to eat—which means deterioration of your overall health.

True, now implants have evolved to replace missing teeth and almost eliminate the need for dentures in some people, but implants are not your natural teeth and do not have those precious nerve fibers judging forces applied to teeth to protect them. Like hip replacements, tooth replacements become expensive and are not the real thing, nor do they last forever. They must be replaced at some future date.

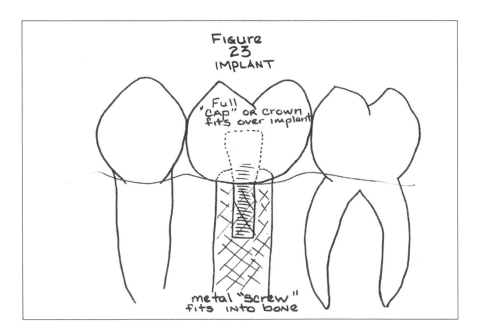

Figure 23
IMPLANT

Full "CAP" or crown fits over implant

metal "screw" fits into bone

Trust the right doctors and care providers, and you can maintain a healthy mouth (and body) for a lifetime.

So what does all this mean, and how can you decide if your provider is right or wrong? What is right or wrong?

Only you can answer these questions, but here are a few guidelines.

First, most people either really love their dentist (or medical physician or pharmacist) or they really hate them. The reasons vary, and they are irrelevant. If you love your dentist, stay there. You obviously feel comfortable to ask all the necessary questions and get all the answers to maintain health, and you are doing what you need to maintain it. Or, you don't really care to hear it and spend all that money, and he never says anything, so why rock the boat? After all, he's kept these remaining teeth in your mouth quite a while now. If you are this type of patient, I doubt you've read this far. So, those of you still with me here, let's get your spies in order.

Most health care providers genuinely want the best for all their patients. Like in all professions, there are some poor providers, but overall there is way too much stress in the health-care field for anyone to stay in it if they genuinely do not care. We do want you to get healthy. We do want you to have the best treatment to stay healthy. We do want you to understand your options and make the right decisions for your life. But sometimes personalities conflict, or some other reason may cause discontent with your provider.

If that's the case, then change. Really. Even doctors prefer you seek care elsewhere if you truly feel uncomfortable.

First try talking it out. Maybe the reason you feel left out can easily be reconciled. Maybe not. Maybe you love the doctor but hate the front desk girl. Or hate the doctor but love the hygienist. Your relationship with the hygienist remains important, but the hygienist does not have the diagnostic skills or education level of a doctor. (I was a hygienist for ten years before becoming a doctor. The level of education doctors receive far exceeds hygiene education.) You need a great relationship with your hygienist, but also, and more importantly, with your doctors.

Maybe you never fully understood a treatment and became dissatisfied with the results. Ask.

Ask why you experience the discomfort, whether physical or emotional, and maybe by learning more you'll realize everything is not really as bad as your imagination led you to believe.

Ask why your teeth keep breaking and it seems you need a crown every year. Ask why your gums still bleed even though you do everything possible. Ask questions and get the answers.

And think about yourself. Now that you know the proper way to clean your mouth, are you doing it? Have you informed your doctor about all those herbal supplements and "natural" remedies you started taking? Prior to reading this book you may not have bothered, because what does that have to do with your teeth anyway, right? Now you know how intricately the system connects.

What about the stress you suddenly have going on? Forget to mention it? You have two daughters getting married this year, and your son graduates from law school, and your husband lost his job… Think you're not grinding your teeth? *Huh!* Think again.

You need to take responsibility for informing your providers so they know to pay closer attention to signs they may otherwise miss. Doctors can fix things, but only you can prevent them in the first place. And if you don't ask or inform us, we cannot possibly read your mind and know. (Maybe someday in the futuristic world, but not yet.)

Also, busyness does come into play, as much as I hate to admit this. Many times the health-care system forces less time spent with each person due to such an overloaded patient schedule. Only you can prevent problems, so ask. Regardless of how busy the office is, your doctor should take the time to answer your questions, or at least listen to them and send appropriately educated staff to answer them for you. Get answers.

Now that you brought all these issues to the attention of your provider, how do they respond? Do they take the time to answer your concerns, or tell you not to worry about all that crap you read on the Internet? (I actually had a urologist say that to me once, and when he learned I am a doctor also, he nearly fell over backwards and changed his tune fast. That still did not make me happy, and I refuse to refer patients to him.) Do you have a personal preference for a female or male practitioner? Younger and more freshly educated, or older and more experienced? Only you can decide your comfort zone.

So change doctors.

How do you find a new doctor?

Ask around. Ask family and friends not only who they see, but why they like that office. Dig deep. As a general rule, people love their dentists. Why? Get some answers. Ask what they would like the office to do differently, and why. Ask if they like the cleanliness, the staff, or the doctor personally. What is it they love?

Ask your pharmacist, physician, or nurse who they recommend as a dentist and why, or vice versa. Ask your physician or dentist who they prefer as a doctor (yes, dentists are doctors) or pharmacist (pharmacists have doctorate degrees, too), and why. Your pharmacist, physician, and dentist are your most important spies. They learn everything about you and are responsible for your overall general health, after you.

Did you catch that? *After* you. Again, only you can prevent problems in the first place. The three primary caregivers above fix problems after they occur or help keep an eye out for you, finding anything deviating from your normal baseline and informing you of its presence. You maintain the responsibility for finding and preventing in the first place.

Call the local dental society and give them information about what type of office you seek based on the questions above, as well as letting them know if you seek a male or female practitioner, or whether you prefer an older and experienced or younger and fresher doctor. How far are you willing to travel for your care? In my practice in Chicago I had patients living in Arizona, Boston, and New York. They kept their twice-annual visits, and if we found treatment necessities, we worked in a time while they were still in the city to get it done. You don't need to travel that far, but you do need to build a strong relationship with the people responsible for maintaining your life along with you, and it pays to stay with them.

The dental society can steer you to a few practices meeting your specific requirements. Then set up a visit with each office before deciding which one to call your home. Our office offers a free "Meet and Greet" appointment for prospective patients. They get to meet my staff, tour my office and sterilization area, and meet me. If the office appeals to them, they set up an appointment for a consultation. If not, they move on without incurring any cost.

During the consultation appointment, ask the doctor if they belong to organized dental groups, and why or why not. For example, the Academy of General Dentistry members must average twenty-five continuing education courses annually to maintain membership, showing a commitment to bettering their knowledge for the best treatment for patients. (Most AGD members average about forty hours annually, and most states only require eighteen to twenty-one hours to maintain a license.)

American Dental Association members gain constant information on local, state, and national updates in legislation, science, and events in the changing world of dental and health care. Ask the provider how much continuing education they take each year and how much their team participates in. Ask about their commitment to excellence for you and how they feel about using a team approach to your health care. A team approach means the doctors contact each other whenever needed or by your request, and you become an active participant taking responsibility for your care.

Ask how they manage emergencies, especially after hours. Ask what procedures stay in-house and which they refer out. I hate doing root canals. I am a visual person, and not being able to see what I am doing grates on me. It's better for a patient in my practice needing a root canal to be seen by a doctor who loves working with the strict tactile sense needed for root canals, and it's better for me not to stress out about doing a procedure you are already stressed to be having done!

If you are comfortable, treated personally, and cared for as a person, if the staff shakes hands with you and introduces themselves, if they look you in the eye as they speak with you and listen to your concerns, if they know that your time is considered valuable, if the cleanliness and professionalism you experience meet your criteria, and if your name isn't just hollered out a peep hole from the door, you have met your spies.

Your first appointment to establish you as a patient in a dental (and medical) office may entail a detailed full medical and social history (which you now know are very relevant to "just" the teeth), getting updated X-rays (we need to see the bone and underlying parts of the teeth not visible in the mouth), an examination of your mouth, bite, and surrounding structures (neck, muscles, glands, and TMJ) and perhaps photographs and study impressions for gathering baseline data to fully understand where your health is from the first meeting. This baseline gives information on many levels, like my patient with the lemon water incident. I knew he had meticulous hygiene habits. I knew his baseline. Where did all these new cavities come from? What changed?

The baseline data becomes the cornerstone to your continued care. If your first visit is for an emergency or you "just want a cleaning" before any knowledge is shared and accepted, you are not using the highest intelligence to achieve great results. You are not being a great general. Problems will break down your surveillance and lead to destruction.

Establish a baseline from which your providers can work.

Usually the next step requires getting disease under control, then any rehabilitation or restructuring with the goal of regaining optimal health. You need spies here because you cannot see inside your own mouth clearly and accurately, nor can you be sure of whether something is normal or not. Many times a patient comes to me panicking about a giant lump on the roof of their mouth. A palatal torus cannot be found in all mouths, but it occurs so often we call it an anomaly, something that is abnormally normal. I'm using a play on words here, but the point is that we learned all the abnormalities and normal structures that can and do occur. You haven't. Spies need reconnaissance, and generals need spies. We are your spies. Let us look, observe, study, and know what the battlefield (your mouth) looks like.

A general dentist in the United States graduates from an accredited university, then spends four years in an accredited dental school concentrating on learning the whole body system and how the teeth relate and function within it, as well as how to help patients keep their teeth healthy and strong. Dentists also learn all the diseases inhabiting a body and the pharmaceutical drugs to treat these diseases. Twice during the curriculum (sophomore year and senior year), students must pass rigorous board examinations testing all this knowledge and the hands-on technical skills.

Upon graduation from dental school, they receive either a DDS (Doctorate of Dental Surgery) or DMD (Doctorate of Medical Dentistry) degree, which today have no difference in education requirements. The general practicing dentist is your primary care physician of the mouth, treating all ages and all oral conditions. The care given provides over sixteen areas of expertise ranging from cosmetics, implants (tooth replacements), root canals, pediatrics (child care), surgery (gums and all areas of the mouth, including pulling teeth), cleanings, periodontics (care of the gums), TMJ treatments, nutrition and tobacco counseling, routine fillings, full mouth reconstruction, and even Botox injections—as dentists know the facial muscles better than most other specialties of the health care professionals. The dentist is the mouth specialist. Now that you know the mouth influences every part of the body, you want your provider keeping up on education, as that information is a lot to remember and constantly changing as more research develops with cancer treatments, medications, and tooth replacement therapies.

I have dealt with cancer specialists telling my patient who was recently diagnosed with cancer to avoid seeing the dentist until their cancer treatments are completed, because of the mouth sores they will get. The line of thought here is: He is the cancer specialist, and dentists are the mouth specialists. Let him treat the cancer and the dentist treat the mouth. But as the mouth specialists, we may be able to prevent those mouth sores in the first place.

Whether you seek a dentist, naturopathic or allopathic physician, or pharmacist, the primary caregiver oversees your health concerns and should be aware of what the entire team of providers is working on in their separate specialties for your one body. You should strive to maintain open communication between all health providers, including medications and supplements you take. All your doctors, and you, should always receive copies of your lab results so everyone knows your baseline standard of health. This way, changes can be tracked readily. When you have your annual blood test done, don't hesitate to send a copy to your dentist. I am tickled pink to know this information about some patients, as it sometimes helps explain things I had no explanation for. Your spies can keep you informed on areas you do not have the privilege to see or know about on your own.

Treat your spies well because good spies win wars.

"Every tooth in a man's head is more valuable than a diamond."
MIGUEL DE CERVANTES: <u>DON QUIXOTE</u>

CHAPTER 8

· · · · · · · · · · · · · · · · · · ·

WINNING THE WAR

*"Everyone thinks of changing the world but
no one thinks of changing himself."*
LEO TOLSTOY

Keeping Your Teeth for a Lifetime

Sun Tzu let it be known that all men can see the tactics used to conquer, but no man can see the strategy out of which victory is evolved. Setting your strategies and employing proper tactics involves forethought and work. You have now learned why you always had tooth problems and why your gums have always bled. You could have hired the wrong spies or delayed moving forward when the time to attack presented itself. You may have separated your soldiers from their unit or depleted your energy sources. Or, you never understood the plans.

Make your corrections from this book and notice over the next few years the overall changes in your mood, health, and checkup appointments. Of course it is better to do all the treatment at once, but that makes it difficult to stay the course. Take baby steps. Set out a strategy to regain complete optimal health.

Make a plan for your health recovery. Make one small change at a time until you master that change, and then make the next one. Change the way you hold your toothbrush and get more plaque off. Master that, then floss the six lower incisors and canines every single day. The saliva glands under the tongue and the tiny size of the teeth make the plaque buildup in that area occur rapidly.

Master flossing the lower incisors and canines so that every dental cleaning appointment you have absolutely no tartar in there. Then floss the rest of your teeth. By that time, you should feel the plaque buildup in the rest of your mouth and *want* to floss!

Imagine that, wanting to floss all your teeth every day! Bet you can hardly wait!

Gradually add more vegetables to your diet until you no longer crave the crap you've been scarfing down. Be mindful of your chewing, and swallow well-chewed mush. Soon you will notice how much better you feel, possibly even clear up that IBS or gluten intolerance—and all you've done is change how you think about eating, using food as energy.

Check in with your spies regularly, and gain new insight to the world within you. Be aware of the enemies within and maintain a readiness to conquer them.

One step at a time, one day at a time, always move forward. Buddha once said, "If you only travel on sunny days, you'll never reach your destination."

Keep traveling forward, little by little. Pay attention to the battle, plan your strategies, and employ the proper tactics, and eventually you will win this war—dying healthy and with all your own teeth in your mouth!

CONCLUSION

· · · · · · · · · · · · · · · · · · · ·

*"It's supposed to be a professional secret but I'll tell you anyway.
We doctors do nothing. We are at best when we give the doctor
who resides within each patient a chance to go to work."*
ALBERT SCHWEITZER MD

You don't know what you don't know.

Words spoken to me decades ago led me on a quest to constantly know more. All these years later, I constantly strive to learn new things.

Teaching others forces me to learn more than I do as a student. In writing this book for you, even though it comes from more than three decades of studying and practicing the principles and using most of this information daily, I learned so much.

Although I talk about dental health with my patients, I had to learn to translate certain dental principles into plain English to assure that those who knew nothing more about their teeth than "those white things in my smile" would find reason to keep those white things their entire lifetime. I learned how to explain the most complex joint in the body in layman's terms for you, a task so difficult to explain even to dentists.

I learned that not everyone cares about health as much as I do. I hope I made it understandable for those of you in this category, so that now health is a higher priority for you.

I learned how to turn excuses into analogies so you can logically understand more about how your body functions as many systems in a single unit, and why one part never has a concern without affecting other parts.

I had so much fun learning about battlefields, strategy, and spies and using the mouth, even the entire human body, as the battlefield upon which combat occurs daily.

As I stated in the beginning, although this is a lofty goal, I hope to have a practice where the only treatments my patients need are preventive care. I am the spy finding small discrepancies they cannot see or reach, and designing strategies with them to conquer misfortune and converting their mouths back to health.

You are the general of your army, loading up your armamentarium (toothbrush, floss, etc.) to keep the enemy (bacteria, specifically PG and colleagues) at bay, and enlisting your spies to become a force to be reckoned with and cause surrender (from the bacteria).

You want to keep your teeth for a lifetime, but where? In a jar on the table next to your bed, or strong and healthy in your mouth? I wrote this book a little bit tongue-in-cheek (pun intended), but in a no-nonsense way. I hope to have taught you the importance of keeping your teeth in your mouth, where they belong.

I hope now that you have read this book you're developing strategies to win the war for good strong dental health.

I may actually achieve my goal, where all my patients, those I see in my practice and those of you reading this book, have healthy mouths and healthy bodies, and my work becomes preventive care only.

Thank you!

Fight on, soldier. Fight on!

ABOUT THE AUTHOR

• • • • • • • • • • • • • • • • • • •

"The goal of my practice is simply to help my patients retain their teeth all of their lives if possible. In maximum comfort, function, health, and esthetics. And to accomplish this appropriately."
L.D. PANKEY, DDS

Dr. Margaret McMillan began studying dental hygiene in 1977. In 1987, she graduated from Northwestern University Dental School with honors. Her never-ending thirst for knowledge led her to become a Fellow in the Academy of General Dentistry by 1996 and a Master Dentist of the Academy in 2006—a feat only 2 percent of all doctors achieve.

Dr. McMillan grew up on the south side of Chicago and now lives with her husband, Slava Kuznetsov, a composer from Siberia, in Zillah, Washington, along with a menagerie of dogs, cats, and other animals. Besides her dental practice, she and Slava own an artist and wellness retreat. In addition to all her achievements in dentistry, she earned certification as a yoga instructor, fitness trainer, and Master Reiki healer. Their retreat offers creativity and health coaching for mind, body, and spirit, concentrating on overall health and wellness.

Dr. McMillan is currently working on her next book, *The Art of War on Diabetes*.

Dr. McMillan can be reached in the following ways:
www.margaretmcmillan.com   drmcmillan@yahoo.com
www.aramistique.com   aramistique@yahoo.com
(509) 829-5006

RESOURCES

. . . .

Here is a list of resources you can check out to gain more information specific to your health interests.

The Art of War by Sun Tzu, translated into English by Lionel Giles, Dell Publishing, in public domain

The Academy of General Dentistry, www.agd.org

The American Dental Association, www.ada.org

The Pankey Institute for Higher Dental Learning, Key Biscayne, Florida www.pankey.org

The Dawson Academy for Higher Dental Learning, St. Petersburg, Florida www.thedawsonacademy.com

www.dentalcare.com

www.crestprohealth.com

www.colgate.com

www.healthmagazine.com

www.healthylivingmagazine.us

www.womanshealthmagazine.com

www.menshealthmagazine.com

The following publications by Dr. Andrew Weil:
www.drweil.com; *8 Weeks to Optimal Health*, Knopf Publishing, 2001; *Eating Well for Optimal Health*, William Morrow Publishing, 2001; *Spontaneous Healing—How to Discover and Enhance Your Body's Natural Ability to Heal Itself*, Ballantine Books, 1996

The Doctor's Book of Home Remedies by *Prevention* magazine editors, www.preventionmagazine.com

Consumer Reports magazine, www.consumerreportshealth.com